Coping with Gout

Christine Craggs-Hinton, mother of three, followed a career in the civil service until, in 1991, she developed fibromyalgia, a chronic pain condition. Christine took up writing for therapeutic reasons, and has in the past few years produced more than a dozen books for Sheldon Press, including *Living with Fibromyalgia, The Chronic Fatigue Healing Diet, Coping Successfully with Psoriasis* and *How to Lower Your Blood Pressure*. Since moving to the Canary Islands, where she is the resident agony aunt for a local paper, she has also taken up fiction writing.

Overcoming Common Problems Series

Selected titles

A full list of titles is available from Sheldon Press,
36 Causton Street, London SW1P 4ST and on our website at
www.sheldonpress.co.uk

Overcoming Common Problems Series

Overcoming Common Problems Series

Overcoming Common Problems

Coping with Gout

Second edition

CHRISTINE CRAGGS-HINTON

sheldon **PRESS**

First published in Great Britain in 2004

Sheldon Press
36 Causton Street
London SW1P 4ST
www.sheldonpress.co.uk

Reprinted twice
Second edition published 2010

British Library Cataloguing-in-Publication Data
A catalogue record for this book is available from the British Library

ISBN 978–1–84709–148–2

1 3 5 7 9 10 8 6 4 2

Typeset by Fakenham Photosetting Ltd, Fakenham, Norfolk
Printed in Great Britain by Ashford Colour Press

Produced on paper from sustainable forests

Contents

Note to the reader

This book is intended as a guide to help lower your risk of further episodes of gout, enabling you to lead a more fulfilling life. It is not a medical book and it is not intended to replace advice from your doctor. If you think you have gout and have not consulted your doctor, please do so.

Introduction

For centuries, gout was known as 'the disease of kings and plenty' – the result of overindulgence in food and drink. Indeed, in the seventeenth to nineteenth centuries much fun was poked at the condition by lampoonists, who delighted in ridiculing the wealthier classes. Unfortunately, old notions have lingered on, and even now individuals can face laughter when they reveal their diagnosis. However, this condition can be exceedingly painful, as anyone who suffers from it will confirm. It certainly doesn't warrant merriment.

Despite its having been observed for around two thousand years, the reasoning that gout was a disease of excess long influenced the lack of significant progress into its causes and treatment. It's only fortunate that in the last hundred years great advances have been made, with experts finally recognizing that the condition is not necessarily – however unintentional – the individual's 'own fault'.

So what have we learned? Well, we now know that it is the people with raised levels of uric acid in their bodies – uric acid being a waste product – who are predisposed to developing gout. Excess uric acid is usually eliminated from the body in the urine, but a variety of things can prevent this from happening. Poor kidney function is a major factor in uric acid build-up as their main task is to remove waste products from the blood and excrete them in the urine.

Other predisposing factors include having a family history of gout, being overweight, taking certain medications or having high blood pressure. It is also possible for the body to pump out unnaturally high levels of uric acid – usually as a result of drinking too much alcohol or eating foods with a high purine content. Purines are substances commonly found in red meat, offal, certain seafood and certain vegetables, as discussed in this book.

As a result of recent research, we now know that it's possible to correct gout in some people and keep it under control in others. There is no magic potion, however. Coping successfully with gout depends largely on the individual working closely with their doctor and being committed to making certain diet and lifestyle changes. The recommended changes are described in this book, along with information about natural remedies, medications and complementary therapies. There is even a chapter on emotional help.

> People wish their enemies dead – but I do not.
> I say give them the gout, give them the stone!
>
> (Lady Mary Wortley Montagu,
> in a letter to Horace Walpole)

1
What is gout?

Gout – sometimes referred to as *podagra* or acute gouty arthritis – is an acute form of arthritis which usually affects the joints. The condition commonly arises in intermittent 'attacks' and is characterized by the following symptoms:

• tenderness and pain (often severe)
• inflammation
• swelling
• reddening
• a mild fever.

An attack of acute gout will normally come on suddenly and swiftly, generally overnight. The affected area will start to feel hot and the skin will become red and appear shiny. Within an hour or so, it may become so painful that even the bedclothes start to feel too heavy. In many cases the individual may also develop a mild fever. The term gout is derived from the Latin word *gutta*, which means a drop – probably because it felt like red-hot liquid dropping on to the area concerned. Gout is recognized as being one of the most painful conditions in medicine.

Although gout is usually associated with the base of the big toe, any joint in the body can be affected, and occasionally it can strike at more than one joint at once. Other areas affected can be the heel, ankle, knee, hand, wrist or elbow. However, it is thought that over half of first attacks affect the big toe. The patient will often limp into the doctor's surgery wearing an open-toed sandal, as contact with shoes or socks can intensify the pain.

If left untreated a mild attack may last for a few days, but a severe attack can persist for several weeks, with some residual pain and discomfort for a further few weeks. After the attack, the area typically returns to normal. Unfortunately, though, after an initial attack, there is a 90 per cent chance of further attacks following, becoming more painful each time, causing permanent damage in the joint and affecting other areas. In time, the pain does not resolve itself between flare-ups and the damage becomes more pronounced. Obviously, this can result in severe mobility problems and ensuing depression. However, by making certain diet and lifestyle adjustments (either instead of or in conjunction with prescription medications) the progress of the disease can be halted long before this stage is reached.

Gout can also present itself in one or more of the tendons, in the cartilage or as lumps (known as *tophi*) under the skin. Moreover, the condition can be complicated by the growth of stones (known as *calculi*) in the urinary system. These possible developments are discussed in later pages.

Who gets gout?

According to the UK Gout Society, gout affects approximately 1 per cent of the population, and that number is slowly rising. A recent survey by market analysts Taylor Nelson Sofres found that 3 per cent of the adults questioned had experienced gout at some time in their lives. The condition occurs in adults of both sexes, but is thought to be at least ten times more common in men than in women. Levels of a chemical called uric acid (urate) tend to increase in men at puberty, and because it takes at least 20 years of raised levels to cause the symptoms of gout, men commonly develop it in their late thirties and through their forties. Women typically develop gout in later life, often in their sixties and seventies. According to some experts, oestrogen – the 'female' hormone – protects against raised levels of uric acid, and when oestrogen levels fall during menopause, levels of uric acid begin to build up.

Some research shows, however, that gout is on the increase in women, with the incidence having doubled over the past 20 years. Boston University School of Medicine found that increasing age, obesity, hypertension, alcohol use, and diuretic use are among leading contributors for women. The study found that higher levels of uric acid in the blood increase the gout risk for women.

What causes gout?

Gout is usually linked to raised levels of uric acid in the blood, over an indeterminate period. It gradually forms into crystal-like deposits which irritate the lining of a particular joint. Everyone has some uric acid in their body, but it is generally harmless and eliminated with the urine or faeces. It is only when levels have been higher than normal for a length of time that problems can occur.

What is uric acid (urate)?

Uric acid is another name for metabolic waste – that is, it is a by-product of the chemical processes that occur within the body. This substance is formed in the liver as the body degrades waste products such as old skin cells and substances called purines that are present in some foods (see pp. 4–7 for more information about purines). Such waste products cannot be broken down within the body and so may build up in the blood.

The quantity of uric acid produced each day by the body is largely determined by the amount of skin cells and purines broken down, and the levels of energy used. Both of these things are proportionate to the body size of the individual, with a large person producing more uric acid than a small person. The concentration of uric acid in bodily tissues depends also on the balance between the amount produced by the liver and the amount passed out via the kidneys. The ability of the kidneys to eliminate uric acid is determined, to a great extent, by inherited factors. It can also depend on whether or not the individual has other health problems, including kidney disease.

In a healthy person, approximately two-thirds of the uric acid produced each day is passed out of the body in the form of urine. The remainder moves into the intestine and is broken down and eliminated in the faeces. Any excess uric acid builds up in the bloodstream and is eventually deposited as urate crystals in the small joints and/or soft tissues.

Before the onset of the first gout attack, there is usually a latent period during which levels of uric acid in the blood gradually increase. As there are no symptoms, this period is known as *asymptomatic hyperuricemia* and can last for several years. You may be surprised to learn that 95 per cent of people with asymptomatic hyperuricemia have it indefinitely and it never develops into gout.

How is uric acid (urate) produced in the body?

Many of the foods we eat contain chemicals called purines. Purines are *nucleotides* – that is, they are the basic molecular building blocks of DNA. (DNA is the self-replicating structure that carries our individual genetic information. It is present in every cell in our bodies.) Along with other nucleotides, purines are sources of energy that drive most of our bodily processes.

After digestion, some purines are absorbed by the intestinal mucosa into nucleic acids. The others are rapidly degraded into uric acid. It is when the ability of the kidneys to eliminate uric acid (via the urine) is compromised that raised levels of uric acid occur – a condition known as *hyperuricemia*. 'Hyper' means increased, 'uric' refers to uric acid and 'emia' (sometimes spelt aemia) means blood. Thus hyperuricemia means raised levels of uric acid in the blood.

Raised levels of uric acid can be caused:

• when less uric acid is removed (via the kidneys) from the body than usual;
• when more is produced (by the liver) than normal;
• when both of the above occur.

Ninety per cent of gout cases are caused by under-excretion of uric acid by the kidneys.

Hyperuricemia

In testing for gout, the concentration of uric acid in the blood serum is measured and is a reflection of levels throughout the body. The recommended range of uric acid levels is less than 6 mg per 100 ml; the range of raised levels is 6–9 mg per 100 ml; and high levels are defined as more than 9 mg per 100 ml. Many people without gout have raised levels of uric acid, which is seen as an indication that the condition is liable to develop in them in future. Urate crystals take a long time to accumulate and, as mentioned, may well never develop into gout – in fact about 95 per cent of people with hyperuricemia will remain symptom-free throughout their lives. On the other hand, a large study in the USA revealed that all participants with high concentrations of uric acid developed gout within four years.

In most cases of gout, there is no clear reason for the build-up of uric acid. However, it is known that certain factors can be responsible. These include:

• a high-purine diet
• poor kidney function or kidney disease
• being overweight

- high levels of fats (lipids) in the bloodstream
- high blood pressure (hypertension)
- regular, excessive alcohol consumption, or binge-drinking
- haemorrhages in the gastro-intestinal canal
- the presence of a disease with a high rate of cell turnover – such as psoriasis, leukaemia and cancer of the lymph nodes (lymphoma)
- the use of certain medications
- dehydration
- inheritance of certain genes, making the person susceptible to gout
- trauma from injury of some kind, causing extensive tissue destruction
- major surgery.

Because gout was uncommon during and immediately after the First and Second World Wars, there is a strong case for its still being referred to as 'the disease of plenty'. In fact, an acute attack often follows an evening of wining and dining or a holiday where restraint is set aside. The disorder is manifest typically in the overweight, hypertensive, overindulgent middle-aged or elderly male.

A high-purine diet

Gout arises from the normal breakdown of our own DNA into nucleic acids, then into purines, then into uric acid. This process accounts for some of the uric acid in our bodies, but a proportion of our purines comes from our diets as well – and again these purines are broken down into uric acid. Unfortunately, a diet that is high in purines burdens the kidneys with a large load for excretion. The same is the case in some individuals who eat a large amount of food containing only a moderate amount of purines. The kidneys may not always be able to cope, hence the raised levels of uric acid.

Purines come from the nuclei of cells, not only of animals but also of plants. The foods that contain purines are: all meats, poultry and seafood, asparagus, mushrooms, dried peas and beans, lentils, soya, spinach and yeast. With meat, a good rule of thumb is that eating any part that has worked hard during its life is more likely to lead to raised levels of uric acid – liver and kidneys, for example. Similarly, chicken breast meat is lower in purines than the legs on which the bird ran about. Active fish, such as sardines and salmon, contain more purines than less lively fish such as plaice and flounder. Regarding alcohol, a product of yeast fermentation, the picture is a little more complex. Most alcoholic drinks contain only small amounts of purine, but its breakdown within the body causes uric acid levels in the blood to rise.

For people who consume moderate amounts of purine foods, cutting them out for five to seven days can significantly reduce levels of uric acid, as shown in a study in 1997.[1] People who are used to eating large amounts of purine foods can find by eliminating them for a few days that their uric acid levels fall even more. (There is more information about diet in Chapter 3.) A urine test after a week of elimination will show the extent of benefit that might be achieved from modifying the diet. If uric acid levels remain unchanged, purine intake is not the real problem. Moderate to high purine consumption is thought to account for only 15 per cent of cases of gout.

Poor kidney function or kidney disease

Any disorder of the kidney reduces its ability to filter and eliminate uric acid. Whether kidney disease is likely to produce hyperuricemia, however, depends to some extent on the concentration of uric acid in the blood prior to the onset of the disease. If the concentration was low and there was only a modest rise with the onset of kidney disease, levels may remain within the normal range. If concentration was towards the upper end of normal, kidney disease is likely to lead to the development of hyperuricemia.

In cases where kidney disease is resolved and function returns to normal, uric acid levels may also return to normal. Of course, this depends also on the weight of the individual, their diet, alcohol intake and many other things.

Diseases of the kidney that can produce hyperuricemia are polycystic kidney disease, kidney disease due to lead poisoning in childhood and kidney disease due to excessive consumption of painkillers. Kidney disease in gout needs the specialized training of a rheumatologist.

Being overweight

Studies have shown that people who are overweight are more likely to have raised levels of uric acid in their blood than people who are not. In fact, being overweight is recognized as the most common cause of hyperuricemia. When weight is lost, the ability of the kidneys to pass out uric acid has been shown to improve. Also, uric acid in the blood reduces and high blood pressure can moderate. It can be seen, then, that weight has a significant impact on hyperuricemia and ultimately gout.

High levels of fats (lipids) in the bloodstream

The levels of fats in the blood are no higher in people with gout than in people with other diseases. However, it is thought that approximately half of the gout population have a condition called *hypertriglyceridemia* – raised levels of triglycerides in the blood (triglycerides are made up of glycerol and fatty acids). The main causes of raised triglyceride concentration in the blood are being overweight (eating a diet that is high in fats) and alcohol consumption, both of which are capable of raising levels of uric acid. Unfortunately, hypertriglyceridemia can lead to diabetes and heart disease, so should really be tackled. Correction of the cause of hypertriglyceridemia can lower levels of uric acid in the blood.

High blood pressure (hypertension)

Hypertension can reduce the kidney's ability to eliminate uric acid, which can in itself lead to hyperuricemia. Kidney disease can also be the cause of high blood pressure, which obviously compounds the situation. In addition, most of the diuretics (water tablets) prescribed to treat hypertension – furosemide and chlorothiazide for example – can lead to the development of hyperuricemia as a side effect. Spironolactone is the only diuretic that doesn't. ACE (angiotensin converting enzyme) inhibitors often successfully reduce high blood pressure, which in turn causes a lowering in levels of uric acid.

In people who are overweight, losing weight can also have the happy side effect of reducing high blood pressure. People with gout would be best advised to have their blood pressure taken at least once a year.

Regular, excessive alcohol consumption

There is a clear association between alcohol consumption and hyperuricemia. In fact after body weight it has the strongest correlation with levels of uric acid in the blood. Studies have shown higher than average concentrations of uric acid in individuals who drink more than two units of alcohol on a regular basis. They have also shown significant drops in concentration when the person cuts down on the amount they drink.

The presence of certain diseases

Any disease in which there is a rapid breakdown and turnover of bodily cells will raise levels of uric acid in the blood. In severe psoriasis, for example, the turnover of skin cells is much faster than normal. This has an effect on the degradation of purines, on the levels of uric acid produced and on the elimination of uric acid by the kidneys. Increased turnover of the bone marrow, in leukaemia and glandular fever for example, can also raise levels of uric acid.

Overweight diabetics with insulin resistance are at risk of developing hypertriglyceridemia (see p. 8) and hyperuricemia because their uric acid is not effectively excreted by the kidneys. (Insulin resistance means the cells have difficulty converting glucose to energy. In an effort to compensate, the pancreas produces more insulin, which creates higher circulating levels of insulin than normal.) The result is often abnormal cholesterol and lipid levels, as well as weight gain. Raised levels of uric acid can also result from hypothyroidism (abnormally low activity of the thyroid gland) and disorders of the parathyroid glands (four small glands located behind the thyroid gland).

The use of certain medications

Diuretics (water tablets) prescribed for high blood pressure can lead to hyperuricemia. Also, chemotherapy drugs used to treat cancer often promote hyperuricemia due to the cell destruction they cause. Aspirin, in low doses, has the effect of reducing the excretion of uric acid, but in high doses it increases elimination. Aspirin should, therefore, be avoided if you suffer from gout. Because some other medications can cause hyperuricemia, check with your doctor to see if they can be the cause of your gout. An alternative medication may be available. If gout is the result of diuretic medication, stopping the diuretic may be possible and all that is required to return uric acid levels to normal.

Inheritance of certain genes

The genes a person inherits can promote either the overproduction or underproduction of uric acid. Small structural defects in the genetic code can affect the control mechanisms for the formation of uric acid, meaning the body produces an abnormally large amount of purine, the precursor to uric acid. The defective gene is located on the X chromosome, which relates to the male. As a result, only males suffer this particular defect, but it can be passed down by a female carrier who herself will either be mildly affected by hyperuricemia or completely normal. Alternatively, the genetic defect can arise spontaneously and there may be no other family members affected.

The ability of the kidneys to eliminate uric acid can also be passed down through families. The average rate of uric acid clearance is 10 ml per minute, the range being between 5 and 15 ml per minute. Those who inherit a clearance rate of only 5 or 6 ml per minute will obviously have much more difficulty eliminating a uric acid load than those who inherit a rate of 14 to 15 ml per minute. Apart from an inherited poor ability to excrete uric acid, the kidney is likely to be normal in all other respects.

Arthritis Research UK is sponsoring research to find out more about the underlying chemical and genetic processes that cause gout and also to search for more effective drugs to treat the disease. Much other research is under way.

When hyperuricemia is present

Hyperuricemia is the state of having raised levels of uric acid in the blood. Over a long period, the uric acid may become so concentrated that it can no longer stay dissolved, and tiny needle-like urate crystals accumulate in the synovial fluid of the joints (the thick lubricating liquid that is secreted into the joint). These urate crystals may, in turn, be present for several years without causing problems. Any of the following events may trigger an attack, however:

- an injury to the joint
- surgery
- illness
- an infection
- drinking too much alcohol

- increasing consumption of purine foods
- starvation
- dehydration
- increased stress
- use of drugs such as thiazides or, ironically, allopurinol, a long-term gout medication, when first used to lower uric acid levels.

Where gout is concerned, there are a few exceptions to the rule. For instance, some people have high levels of circulating uric acid, but this is not accompanied by crystal formation and they do not experience gout. Also, rarely, some people with normal levels of uric acid do suffer from gout. In the main, though, the higher the level of uric acid, the greater the chance that crystals will form and be triggered into gout.

Topheous gout

In the case of an untreated sufferer who over a period of approximately ten years has experienced intermittent attacks of acute gout, a more chronic arthritis slowly develops in which symptoms will not completely resolve between attacks. The urate crystals responsible for acute attacks – which are generally only visible under a microscope – collect together beneath the skin to form a lump called a tophus. Tophi typically appear at the rim of the ear (where they are seen as small firm nodules), in the upper surfaces of the fingers, hands and feet and in the forearms and Achilles tendons. They can even grow in the kidney, severely compromising its filtering mechanisms (see p. 13).

Topheous gout commonly causes deformity and joint immobility. In fact in the days before treatment was available, tophi could grow larger than a golf ball – particularly on the hands and feet – and render the individual unable to function.

The tophi might even discharge a white chalky substance. (It is said that this was once used by some teachers to write on blackboards – what better example could there be of the grossness of gout in the past!) Furthermore, tophi would often become ulcerated and discharge blood and pus – and, of course, in this state they would be exceedingly painful. Thanks to modern medicines and knowledge about management techniques, today very few sufferers need be familiar with these extreme symptoms of the disease: only 15 per cent have tophi at all (compared with 50 per cent prior to the widespread use of medications that lower uric acid levels), and those who do will be prescribed lifelong preventative medication that generally results in the tophi being reabsorbed into the body (see Chapter 2).

In other cases, tophi may drain spontaneously and become infected, further damaging the nearby joint. In elderly women who develop gout after taking diuretics or who suffer compromised kidney function, tophi may appear without previous history of acute gouty attacks. Also, a very rapid development of widespread tophi may occur in kidney and heart transplant patients who are treated with cyclosporine medication.

Topheous gout and kidney disease

When, in the past, no treatment was available for gout, tophi regularly formed in the body of the kidney and urate crystals in the collecting tubes. The cellular changes at the site of the tophi often led to kidney disease – and one result of that is high blood pressure. Of course, high blood pressure has always carried risks of its own, such as heart disease and further kidney disease. Kidney failure might eventually result. Fortunately, we now have medications that can generally prevent this state of affairs arising.

Kidney stones

The kidneys are highly implicated in gout because:

- when hyperuricemia is present, raised amounts of uric acid pass through the kidneys prior to being eliminated from the body, and
- the kidneys work hard to concentrate all the uric acid passing through them.

Because high levels of uric acid pass through the kidneys, tiny crystals of urate can collect together, accumulating into 'stones' that may reach more than 2.5 cm (1 inch) in diameter. In fact, experts believe that up to 40 per cent of gout patients have suffered a bout of renal colic due to the formation of a small stone (*calculus*) within the kidney or urinary tract. When stones remain in the kidney, a dull pain is a common symptom. However, when stones form in the ureters – the tubes that connect the kidneys to the bladder – the flow of urine can be blocked. A common symptom of this is blood in the urine – but sometimes the blood is not visible to the naked eye.

Urine analysis can show white blood cells, after which the patient may be sent for an X-ray or ultrasound scan. Kidney stones can be broken up by ultrasound waves and passed out with the urine, or extracted surgically. However, if levels of uric acid in the blood remain constant, further stones are likely to form.

Kidney stones can cause alarming symptoms. If you notice blood in your urine or start experiencing a constant dull or severe colicky pain in the kidney or groin area, you should visit your doctor immediately.

Paediatric gout

Gout is usually associated with the middle-aged male. Few people are aware that hyperuricemia can occur in individuals of any age. Even young children can develop the condition. In such cases the cause is generally a genetic purine and pyramidine enzyme deficiency. Purines and pyramidines are the building blocks of DNA (see p. 4). Like purines, pyramidines are broken down in the body by a specific enzyme. The first indications of problems may be crystals on the nappy or, in older children, in the urine. The medical term for paediatric gout is familial juvenile hyperuricemia nephropathy (FJHN); it was first described in 1962.

Recent studies have shown that some defects involving purine and pyramidine synthesis are genetic and thus could be seen in people of all ages and both sexes. If not treated adequately, disorders of purine and pyramidine synthesis can deteriorate so that ultimately dialysis is required. Indications of gout in children or adolescents should always be investigated as a matter of urgency.

Pseudogout

Gout-like attacks of pain, stiffness and swelling can be caused by deposits of calcium pyrophosphate crystals within the joints. This is called pseudogout, a form of arthritis which generally strikes at the elderly and immobile. Pseudogout is similar to gout and usually diagnosed when the doctor removes some fluid from a swollen joint with a needle and examines it under a microscope. If urate crystals are observed, the problem is gout, whereas if calcium phosphate crystals are observed, the problem is pseudogout.

The joints most commonly affected in pseudogout are the elbows, wrists, ankles, knees, fingers and toes, but the shoulder and hip joints are sometimes involved. The condition often occurs in more than one area at once. In contrast, gout normally arises in a single joint, usually the base of the big toe.

Pseudogout can respond well to steroid injections and anti-inflammatory medication. However, it is important that the distinction between this type of arthritis and gout be made, as without the right treatment pseudogout can cause permanent joint damage.

There is no known way to prevent this disorder as its cause is unknown.

2
Getting help from your doctor

If you think you are suffering from gout, it is important to secure a diagnosis as early as possible. Gout is one of the easiest forms of arthritis to treat. Remember that forming a close relationship with your doctor will be of benefit to you both – you will feel supported and understood and your doctor will have a better idea of the most suitable treatment options.

Preparing to see your doctor

If you are reading this book, you probably either suspect you have gout or you already have a diagnosis. For those who suspect, it may be helpful to know the official diagnostic criteria.

Diagnostic criteria

The American College of Rheumatology has defined the official criteria for the diagnosis of gout. Six or more of the following 11 criteria should be met to give a diagnosis:

• You must have suffered more than one attack of acute pain in a joint.
• Maximum inflammation must develop within one day.
• You must have suffered at least one attack of oligoarthritis – a type of arthritis that affects children, linked with an eye disease called chronic iridocyclitis.
• Redness must be observed over the affected joint.
• The big-toe joint must be painful and/or swollen.
• Your first attack must be on the joint of one big toe, not on the joint of both big toes.

- An attack must be on the joints of only one ankle.
- There must be one or more tophi present.
- You must have hyperuricemia (raised levels of uric acid in the blood – see Chapter 1).
- You must have asymmetrical swelling within an affected joint on X-ray.
- There must be complete termination of an attack.

Be prepared for your doctor's questions

Your doctor's role is to look at your symptoms, ask a few questions, then attempt to fit the pieces together. Since certain other kinds of arthritis can mimic a gout attack – particularly acute septic arthritis or pseudogout – it is important that the right diagnosis be made. This also applies where an individual presents with a hot, painful and swollen toe, for example, as it could initially be taken for infection.

To properly assess your condition, your doctor may ask a series of questions. They are likely to include the following:

- Which areas of the body are involved?
- When did you first notice there was a problem?
- Did the pain come on suddenly or gradually?
- Was the pain worse during daytime or at night?
- Was the area hot, red and swollen?
- Did you experience other symptoms, such as fever, general achiness, loss of appetite, at the time the area became painful?
- Have you noticed lumps under your skin, especially on the ridge of the outer ear, the fingers, elbows, toes or around the Achilles tendon (which connects the heel bone to the lower leg)?
- Have you ever had kidney stones?
- Does anyone in your family suffer from gout?

Give as much information as possible

To help point your doctor in the right direction, you should offer as much information as you can. Some details may be embarrassing, but they really should be disclosed.

• Your doctor must be reminded of any other illnesses you may have because gout can be associated with other health problems, for example kidney disease, high blood pressure, hypothyroidism, polycythaemia and psoriasis.

• You should state whether you were crash dieting or drinking large amounts of alcohol prior to an attack.

• Let your doctor know if you injured the area shortly before an attack. For example, did you stub your toe prior to it becoming swollen and painful?

• Let your doctor know if you had an infection prior to an attack.

• You should state whether you were eating more organ meat, shellfish or other foods high in purines than usual before the attack.

• Your doctor should also be reminded of any medications you take, as certain ones can trigger a gout attack. Examples are diuretics (water tablets) and low-dose aspirin.

Normally, doctors can diagnose gout on physical examination during an acute attack, combined with the individual's medical history. The definitive diagnosis of gout is dependent on finding uric acid crystals in the joint fluid during an attack (*arthrocentesis* – see p. 21). Doctors can also administer a test, discussed in the next section, that measures the levels of uric acid in the blood. However, although uric acid levels are usually raised in individuals with gout, these levels alone are often misleading and may on measurement be normal or even low. The presence of raised levels of uric acid (hyperuricemia) increases the likelihood of the problem being gout. The development of tophi – often seen as small nodules on the ear – can confirm the diagnosis.

The blood test

In the blood test to measure levels of uric acid, blood is drawn from a vein or capillary. The laboratory then centrifuges the blood to separate the serum from the cells and the uric acid test is performed on the serum.

Preparing for the blood test

Your doctor may ask you to fast for four hours prior to the test. You may also be advised to stop taking any drugs that increase levels of uric acid. These include:

- aspirin
- caffeine
- alcohol
- diuretics (water tablets, such as Diamox, Burinex and Lasix)
- ascorbic acid (vitamin C tablets)
- diazoxide
- ethambutol
- methyldopa
- phenothiazines
- epinephrine
- cisplatin
- vincristine.

Drugs that can decrease uric acid measurements should also, ideally, be temporarily discontinued prior to the test, with the backing of your doctor. These include:

- high-dose aspirin
- allopurinol
- clofibrate
- corticosteroids
- azathioprine
- guafenesin

- probenecid
- warfarin.

The laboratory should be notified if you have recently undergone X-ray testing using contrast dyes. These chemicals increase uric acid levels in urine and decrease them in the blood.

Arthrocentesis

Because the blood test cannot give a definitive diagnosis, your doctor may wish to test the fluid in an affected joint, during an attack. If urate crystals are present the diagnosis is confirmed. This procedure is called arthrocentesis.

What happens during the procedure?

Your doctor will clean the area around the joint and may administer a local anaesthetic. A needle will then be inserted into the joint cavity and synovial fluid will be withdrawn. The doctor may then inject the joint with a drug that reduces inflammation, together with a painkiller. Slight pressure will then be applied to the place where the needle was inserted, and the doctor may wrap a bandage around it. The fluid will then be sent to a laboratory where it will be viewed under a microscope. If urate crystals are found, a diagnosis of gout can be confirmed.

Viewing under a microscope also allows the diagnosis of pseudogout, a similar condition described in Chapter 1, in which the joint pain is caused by deposition of pyrophosphate crystals. Pseudogout often attacks a different range of joints, such as the wrist, shoulder or knee.

What else will the doctor do?

Your doctor will also assess the following:

- your blood pressure;
- your kidney function;

- the levels of lipids (fats) in your blood;
- any existing medication, to gauge whether it has triggered the attack and to ensure it will not interact with any future gout medication;
- the need for X-rays of the affected joints if gout has been present for some time and not treated for any reason.

How is gout treated?

'The gout sir,' replied Mr Weller. 'The gout is a complaint as arises from too much ease and comfort. If you're ever attacked with the gout, sir, just you marry a widder as has got a good loud voice, with a decent notion of usin' it and you'll never have the gout again. It's a capital prescription, sir. I takes it reg'lar, and I can warrant it to drive away any illness as is caused by too much jollity.'

(Charles Dickens, *The Pickwick Papers*)

This quote, funny as it may be, reflects the flawed reasoning that hindered progress in gout treatments for far too long. Fortunately, we have come a long way in the last hundred years and now have a great deal of knowledge about the condition. Currently, its treatment has three aims, which are to:

1 stop the current painful attack;
2 prevent further attacks by tackling the causes (such as high purine intake, drinking too much alcohol, being overweight, eating a high-fat diet);
3 if the above measures are not entirely successful, you can avert further attacks by using long-term preventative medications – joint damage, heart disease, kidney disease can be among the results if gout is not effectively treated.

Medications that treat an acute attack

When an attack of gout takes hold, all you will be able to think about is getting rid of the pain. Consequently, your first step in treatment will focus on reducing the inflammation in the affected area. This should provide you with relief.

Aspirin and its related drugs (salicylates) should be avoided as they can raise uric acid levels and ultimately exacerbate gout. This drug can also cause or worsen bleeding from the stomach. If you take an aspirin tablet each day to reduce the risk of blood clots (and heart attack), speak to your doctor about the possibility of either using an alternative medication or taking an enteric-coated drug with the aspirin to protect your stomach.

Over-the-counter painkillers

Low-dosage codeine combined with paracetamol, available over the counter, can be of help to some people, as can ibuprofen, the only tablet-form non-steroidal anti-inflammatory drug available over the counter. Enteric-coated pills are easier on the stomach.

Prescription non-steroidal anti-inflammatory drugs (NSAIDs)

Acute gouty attacks are usually treated by prescription non-steroidal anti-inflammatory drugs. NSAIDs can calm the process that causes the inflammation, as a result of which the pain and swelling are eased. This family of drugs include naproxen sodium, indometacin and ibuprofen, the latter in a stronger dosage than available over the counter. NSAIDs are often prescribed in double the usual daily dose for the first two days, followed by regular recommended dosing for about one week. Dosing tapers down ultimately to discontinuation.

In the short term, dizziness, indigestion and nausea can arise with NSAID therapy, and prolonged usage can cause stomach and bowel irritation or aggravation of existing kidney disease. Taking NSAIDs with meals can reduce or eliminate these side effects. They should not be used where there is existing kidney disease, a peptic ulcer or inflammatory bowel disease. As there are approximately a hundred medications in this category, your doctor may want to see how you respond to different ones.

Cox-2 inhibitors

In recent years, Cox-2 inhibitors have been introduced. These offer a much lower risk of gastro-intestinal side effects than the traditional NSAIDs, with equal efficacy. In June 2002, the largest trial[2] for the treatment of gout was reported in the *British Medical Journal*, comparing indometacin (an NSAID medication) with the Cox-2 inhibitor etoricoxib. The conclusion was that etoricoxib at 120 mg once a day provided the same rapid, effective relief as indometacin at 50 mg three times a day. This gives doctors another choice for treating acute gout, so that gastro-intestinal upsets become less of a problem.

Colchicine

Colchicine is an old-fashioned gout remedy that was the first to be found effective in the nineteenth century. It is now prescribed mainly in cases where NSAIDs and Cox-2 inhibitors cannot be used. It is also used as a long-term preventative measure, preventing attacks in 80 per cent of patients – usually those with more modest elevations of uric acid in their blood. Unfortunately, this drug is slow to start working and may even cause abdominal pain, nausea and vomiting – but the side effects disappear once the patient stops taking the drug. Colchicine therapy is often given for 12 months or longer after uric acid levels are normalized. It can be prescribed in conjunction with life-long preventative medication that prohibits the build-up of uric acid in the blood.

Corticosteroids

These steroids may be prescribed when NSAIDs, Cox-2 inhibitors and colchicine are inappropriate or have failed, if infection is not present in the joint and only one or two joints are involved. Steroids can be injected directly into the joint or given via mouth. To inject into the joint will be a specialist decision.

Life-long preventative medications

The medications listed above can do nothing to prohibit the build-up of uric acid in the blood, nor can they prevent further acute attacks or stop urate crystals from accumulating in the joints. So what happens if the attacks continue (at the rate of three to four a year), if tophi are present, and if blood tests show that levels of uric acid are building up further? A low-purine diet, weight control, avoidance of alcohol and so on can successfully ward off additional attacks, but these measures don't always work – for example, where kidney disease is present or where medications must be taken for other health problems. Preventative treatment of hyperuricemia is expensive, life-long and carries a risk of toxic side effects. However, when all else fails, this is what your doctor will offer.

Life-long preventative medication works by normalizing levels of uric acid in the blood – in other words, correcting hyperuricemia. As a result, the attacks should stop and any tophi dissolve. (In some cases, medications fail to dissolve the tophi and they must be removed surgically.) The resolution of hyperuricemia has the added bonus of improving the kidney problems that can accompany gout. It also means the prevention of the many complications to which hyperuricemia can lead.

Some people may think, 'Why bother making adjustments to my diet, losing weight, watching what I drink when preventative medications can be used instead?' It must be said that uric acid build-up in the first place is an SOS warning that something is very wrong. If you make no changes, continued weight gain can lead to high blood pressure, heart and lung disease, impaired kidney function, osteoarthritis; excess alcohol consumption can lead to serious liver damage; and a high-fat intake can lead to raised cholesterol levels and heart disease. Nor is this list exhaustive. Changing to healthier habits can prevent the diseases to which less healthy habits often lead. However, it's an unfortunate fact that taking one of the preventative medications can do nothing to improve the actual cause of the problem.

Because preventative medications are expensive and fail to tackle the underlying cause of hyperuricemia, they are generally offered to patients only in the following instances:

- if a health problem not in their control is causing their hyperuricemia – such as kidney disease, psoriasis, hypothyroidism or leukaemia;
- if necessary medications affect uric acid levels in the blood;
- if they suffer from a purine synthesis disorder;
- if they appear to have inherited a genetic overproduction or underproduction of uric acid;
- if they have tried hard to alter their diet, lose weight etc. but have failed;
- if they suffer from an alcohol addiction.

Note that it is vital to let an acute attack settle down before embarking on one of the life-long medications. When the medications are taken erratically, flare-ups of gout are likely to ensue. It is important, therefore, that the medication be taken exactly as prescribed.

Allopurinol

The most common preventative treatment for gout is allopurinol. This drug works by inhibiting an enzyme – xanthine oxidase – that activates the production of uric acid by the liver. Taken daily over a long period, allopurinol will effectively reduce the levels of uric acid, then ensure that levels remain within normal boundaries. The usual starting dose is 100 mg daily, which is increased over the weeks according to the levels of uric acid. Most people end up taking 100–400 mg daily, the maximum daily dose being 800 mg. A dose of 300 mg is effective in 85 per cent of patients, however. The aim is to bring the levels of uric acid in the blood within the recommended range of less than 6 mg per 100 ml.

Allopurinol is known to be relatively safe, but all drugs have potential side effects. In 20 per cent of cases, usually when there is severe kidney disease, patients are hypersensitive to this drug and may develop a nasty rash, dermatitis and possibly liver dysfunction. In this instance, your doctor should be able to offer an alternative preventative medication.

Unfortunately, in some individuals gout attacks can become more frequent on commencement of a life-long treatment. To prevent this, an anti-inflammatory medication or colchicine may also be prescribed during the first three to six months of treatment.

As allopurinol causes a large amount of uric acid to be released into the bloodstream, it should not be taken when a gout attack is in progress. If taken at this time, the situation would undoubtedly worsen.

For this reason, at least a month should elapse after the attack before commencement of this type of treatment. Unfortunately, attacks may still occur in the first months of allopurinol therapy. In some cases, it may take as long as two years for urate crystals to be cleared. Note that if this type of medication is stopped, uric acid will accumulate again in the blood and urate crystals will once more form in the joints.

Uricosuric drugs

Uricosuric drugs such as probenecid and sulfinpyrazone lower the levels of uric acid in the blood by increasing its removal from the body via the kidneys (excretion). Like allopurinol, these drugs are a life-long commitment and need to be strictly adhered to. The side effects related to probenecid and sulfinpyrazone are not common or serious, but there is a risk of uric acid stone formation in the kidney during the initial treatment period, especially in individuals with pre-existing kidney disease. This risk can be minimized by drinking two to three litres of fluid a day.

If the first preventative treatment prescribed causes side effects, your doctor should be able to prescribe another type. Individuals with pre-existing disease or kidney stones should not be prescribed sulfinpyrazone.

The effects of probenecid are blocked by low-dose aspirin. Probenecid also inhibits the effectiveness of the drug heparin.

Where can I get more help and advice?

If you feel you need advice further to that given by your doctor, you can do the following:

- Your pharmacist may be able to offer more information on the lifestyle changes and medications that cause, treat and prevent gout.
- If a certain medication has been prescribed, read the patient information leaflet thoroughly. It will tell you how to use the medication and what benefits or possible side effects you can expect. Bear in mind, though, that many of the side effects listed are likely to be very rare indeed.
- Your doctor can put you in touch with a dietician if you need further assistance in adjusting what you eat. Alternatively, you can get help for any weight problems by joining one of the weight-loss organizations (see the useful addresses section for details).
- If alcohol addiction is a problem, it is recommended that you join a voluntary organization for help and support, such as Alcoholics Anonymous (AA). Your GP may be able to help you and also to advise you about local support groups.

3

Helping yourself

When an acute attack of gout takes hold, all you will want to know is how to ease the pain. Your first step, if you are open to using medication, is to see your doctor and obtain a prescription for one of the non-steroidal anti-inflammatory drugs (NSAIDs), if they are appropriate to your case. It is advisable then to keep a supply of the drug handy for if and when further attacks occur. The following guidelines can help ease the pain and reduce the longevity of the attack:

- Try to rest until the attack is over.
- Increase your fluid intake, trying to drink 3.5 litres (6 pints) of water a day. This should help flush out excess uric acid.
- Eat a bowlful of cherries a day or take cherries in liquid concentrate form, or as powder in capsules (see pp. 30–2). (See the useful addresses section at the back of this book for details of where to purchase these.)
- Use contrast hydrotherapy (alternating three-minute hot compresses with 30-second cold compresses). A warmed-up wheat bag and bag of frozen peas is all that is needed. This treatment can help to break down the urate crystals and resolve the pain faster.
- Assuming you keep non-steroidal anti-inflammatory medications handy (these are effective at killing pain as well as at reducing inflammation), start taking the prescribed dosage – that is, if you wish to use drugs.
- Take belladonna for its anti-inflammatory properties, following the label dosage instructions. Belladonna can be purchased as an over-the-counter homeopathic remedy from

chemists. A constitutional remedy prescribed by an experienced homeopath can help to reduce the likelihood of further attacks.

• Don't eat or drink anything you know is high in purines. If you tend to binge drink at the weekend, avoid it this time.

• As well as avoiding high-purine foods, cut down on red meat and eliminate fried foods.

• Follow a therapeutic diet consisting largely of cheese, milk, eggs and vegetables (excluding cauliflower, asparagus or mushrooms) for the duration of the attack.

• Incorporate more omega 3 into your diet. This helps to reduce pain, inflammation and tissue damage.

• Eat burdock root to help rid the body of uric acid build-up.

If the factors that caused gout in the first place continue, an initial acute attack is likely to be followed, one or two years later, by further attacks. The intervals between flare-ups will become shorter and the attacks themselves more painful and debilitating as deposits of urate crystals form beneath the skin. While medications can be invaluable in treating an acute attack, they are not without side effects. The safest way to treat gout is, if at all possible, to make the necessary adjustments to your diet and lifestyle, so that raised levels of uric acid in the blood revert back to normal. However, if that is not possible for any reason, it is important that you don't be too hard on yourself. Fortunately, preventative medication is also available and it is far better than nothing at all. Stay positive and get on with enjoying a gout-free life.

How cherries can help

In 1950, a letter by Dr Ludwig W. Blau in *Prevention* magazine sparked off much interest in cherries for the treatment of gout. Dr Blau related how eating a bowl of cherries one day led to complete relief from his gout pain.[3] His gout had been so severe that he was confined to a wheelchair – but after polishing off a bowl of cherries the pain in his foot had vanished by the next day. He continued eating a minimum of six cherries every day and was free of pain and able to get out of his wheelchair. Dr Blau's research resulted in many other gout sufferers being helped by the introduction of cherries into their daily diet. Nutritionists believe that this fruit contains an enzyme that helps to break down uric acid and facilitate its excretion from the body.

It is claimed that the *montmorency* cherry is the richest source of health-promoting properties.

Montmorency cherry juice

Ruby red montmorency cherry is high in antioxidants, flavonoids and anthocyanins, which work together to make it an effective treatment for inflammatory conditions such as gout. The montmorency is a variety of sour cherry which is mainly cultivated in the United States, Canada and France. It belongs to the lighter red family of sour cherries, rather than the darker red morello type.

Drinking montmorency cherry juice (which can be purchased in plastic bottles in concentrate form) on a daily basis has been shown in ongoing research to reduce the inflammation of gout and other arthritic conditions like no other fruit or vegetable. In fact, it has been found in research to work in the same way as non-steroidal anti-inflammatory drugs (NSAIDs). Unlike NSAIDs, though, montmorency cherry juice does not cause stomach irritation. Indeed, some researchers claim that this particular type of cherry juice is as effective as aspirin and ibuprofen, but without the risk of stomach ulcers and kidney damage.

I must say that although I don't doubt that montmorency cherries are effective – particularly for treating gout – I would like to see them subjected to more scientifically controlled studies. There have been some very promising studies on rats with arthritis where the cyanidin in cherries was seen to protect against paw inflammation and where antioxidant activity was improved, but we need to see this effect in a range of human studies. The reason this hasn't happened is probably because it's not really feasible to oversee everything eaten and drunk by a human being over several months, whereas it's quite easy to know what a rat in laboratory conditions consumes.

Montmorency cherry juice tastes good, too! If you happen to find it a little tart, try adding a splash of lemonade, dry ginger or some ice-cubes. Each bottle contains 946 ml of concentrate, and the recommended intake is one part concentrate to seven parts water. Pour a two-tablespoon (30 ml) serving of concentrate into a half-pint glass and top up with warm or cold water, depending upon your preference, and drink half a pint (280 ml) daily. The shelf life of montmorency cherry juice is approximately one year in the fridge and 18 months in the freezer – it should always be kept chilled. If the concentrate should crystallize in the freezer, warming it through makes it easier to pour.

Montmorency cherries can also be freeze-dried into powder and packed into capsules, which are easy to take once or twice a day. See the useful addresses section at the back of this book for information on where to purchase this product.

Correcting hyperuricemia

Before hyperuricemia can be tackled, you need to decide what is its probable cause. You can then make efforts to correct it. For example, if you are overweight you can help yourself by following a healthy eating plan that you know you stand a fair chance of continuing for the rest of your life (fad diets are not good for your body and can rarely be maintained). If you drink more than two standard drinks of alcohol a day, you can help yourself by cutting down to healthier levels. If hypertension is also a problem, control of the above factors may have the happy outcome of reducing blood pressure and the need for diuretics (water tablets). A common problem in gout is that several factors may have worked together to cause hyperuricemia. A typical gout sufferer might be an overweight, middle-aged male who is a regular alcohol drinker, eats meat twice a day and has raised levels of fats in his blood (hypertriglyceridemia – see Chapter 1). Since his friends may share the same lifestyle, it can be extremely difficult to find the motivation to make changes. I suggest that if this description fits you, you enlist the support of your family and friends, impressing on them that your gout will worsen if you don't make changes, after which the only alternative would be to take medication for the rest of your life.

When levels of uric acid have been normal for about a year, gout attacks will either become mild and infrequent or disappear altogether.

Stabilizing medication

While you are attempting to normalize levels of uric acid in your blood, you may wish to take medication to reduce the risk of further flare-ups of gout. The best ones are probably colchicine and NSAID drugs (non-steroidal anti-inflammatory drugs) – your doctor will know which is more suitable. Then, as you attempt to correct your hyperuricemia, your blood serum should be checked regularly by your doctor. Knowing that levels of uric acid are falling should give you that extra boost to help you on your way. When you have suffered no attacks of gout for 12 months, it should be safe to come off the medication and continue as you mean to go on.

Note that it is vital to do nothing either to lower or to raise your levels of uric acid during an attack, or while there is persistent gouty inflammation. Any deviation from the norm – barring recommended medication – can worsen the attack.

Important note: It is vital that you wait until an attack is over before you embark on a new medication.

Reducing dietary purines

If you normally consume large amounts of dietary purines, cutting down can have a substantial effect on the levels of uric acid in your blood. On the other hand, if you consume only moderate amounts of purines, your uric acid levels are likely not to alter very much on cutting down. In that case, other factors will have led to your hyperuricemia and you need not alter your intake of purines. Only people who eat large amounts of purines should try to reduce their purine foods. Alternative sources of protein should be added to a low-purine diet. These could include, for example, tofu, tempeh and miso.

Since many protein foods contain purines, it is recommended that your intake of protein should not exceed 100 g (3½ oz) per day. (Many people in whom hyperuricemia is diagnosed eat large amounts of protein in the form of meats – hence the high level of purines.) As a guide, a portion of 100 g of meat contains 25 g protein; of pasta 12 g; of rice 8 g. One thick slice of wholemeal bread contains 3 g protein.

The following is a list of foods showing their relative purine contents:

Very high purine content: Organ meats such as liver, kidney, brains, heart and sweetbreads
Game meats such as rabbit, venison, pheasant, duck, goose and partridge
High purine content: Vegetables such as spinach, asparagus, cauliflower and mushrooms
Chicken
Fish such as herring, sardines, scallops, mackerel, roe, shrimp, mussels and anchovies

Yeast (baker's and brewer's) and yeast extracts (Marmite and Vegemite for example)

Meat extracts and gravies, broth and consommé

Beer, wines and spirits

Dried peas and beans

Moderate purine content: Oatmeal, peas, beans and other legumes, lentils, soya, spinach, tripe and wholemeal (also called wholewheat or wholegrain) bread and pasta

Beef and pork

The foods recommended in gout are:

Breads, especially white bread and crackers (limit intake of higher-fat foods such as muffins, French toast, biscuits and doughnuts, and also of wholemeal bread and biscuits – see above)

Cheese (all kinds in moderation, and preferably low-fat)

Cereals and cereal products (all kinds except oatmeal)

Eggs (in moderation)

Fruit juices (all kinds)

Fruit (all kinds; avocado in limited quantities). (Don't forget that although fruit is good for a gout diet, high amounts can be counter-productive.)

Gelatin

Low-fat meat and fish cooked without oil (a small quantity, no more than 100 g (3½ oz), should be eaten two to three times a week)

Milk (fat-free and low-fat)

Noodles

Nuts (walnuts and hazelnuts in particular)

Oils (all oils, in limited quantities)

Pasta (wholemeal pasta in moderation)
Potatoes (limit intake of higher-fat forms such as chips, potato crisps and creamed potatoes)
Soups (cream soups should be made with low-fat milk)
Vegetables (except spinach, asparagus, cauliflower and mushrooms)
White rice

Eating healthily

Unfortunately, removing purines from the diet is known to cause a drop in uric acid levels of only 15 per cent. Healthy eating can reduce levels further; it will have the happy side effect of weight loss in people who are overweight, and it can reduce levels of triglycerides (fats) in the blood. Healthy eating can also reduce high blood pressure and the risk of both heart and kidney disease. It can therefore be of great benefit in gout.

Although it may be difficult at first to make the recommended changes, the benefit to your overall health will make the effort worthwhile. However, if you find you are unable to make great changes, don't feel guilty or despondent. Small changes are better than no changes at all – they will make a difference. In time, you may find you are able to introduce more changes. Healthy eating advice is given in Chapter 4.

Reducing alcohol consumption

An individual's alcohol consumption is strongly linked to levels of uric acid in the blood, someone drinking moderate to high amounts of alcohol being far more likely to develop hyperuricemia than someone who doesn't drink, or drinks very little. Studies have shown that people who consume more than two units of alcohol on a regular basis have higher than average concentrations of uric acid in the blood. Obviously, some people drink rather more than two units, which has a knock-on effect on levels of uric acid.

Alcohol causes a rise in uric acid levels for the following reasons:

- The metabolism of alcohol creates a chemical called lactate, which reduces the elimination of uric acid by the kidneys.
- Certain properties of alcoholic drinks can pile on the pounds – in males it is generally around the middle – and carrying excess weight has its own links with hyperuricemia.
- Many alcoholic beverages contain purines.

Quite often people don't realize the extent of their alcohol consumption, especially if they tend to drink a glass of wine or two with meals, then more at night socially, or while watching the TV. Drinking beer or lager socially at the pub is a way of life for many people, but they rarely count the number of pints they drink in a week. A person who abstains all week but drinks several pints of beer at the weekend is just as likely to have raised levels of uric acid as someone who drinks beer almost every night. It can be difficult to break what is often a social habit, but it should not be necessary to abstain from alcohol altogether. Try drinking more slowly and replace some of your alcoholic drinks with non-alcoholic ones. Ask your doctor to measure your uric acid levels after cutting down for a while, then decide whether you need to cut down further.

People who binge drink or drink regular amounts of alcohol tend to be overweight. This transpires because of the effect of the kilojoules in the alcohol. Cutting down, therefore, is another great way to lose weight. The government-recommended safety limit for women is no more than 14 units, and for men it is a maximum of 21 units.

So how much drink does it take for you to be an alcoholic? A practical definition of alcoholism is persistent drinking that interferes with your health, legal position, interpersonal

You can measure your alcohol intake by taking note of the following:

Half a pint of normal strength beer, lager or cider equals one unit.
One small (100 ml) glass of wine equals one unit.
A large (175 ml) glass of wine equals two units.
A single (25 ml) measure of spirits equals one unit.
One 275 ml bottle of alcopop (5.5 per cent/volume) equals 1.5 units.

relationships or means of livelihood. In the UK, there are 4 million heavy drinkers, 800,000 problem drinkers and 400,000 dependent drinkers, or alcoholics.

Your answers to these questions may help you to decide whether or not you are addicted to alcohol:

- Do you regularly drink more than you intended?
- Do you crave drink for much of the time?
- Do you drink to escape worries or troubles?
- Do you feel guilty about your drinking?
- Is your drinking causing a problem in any area of your life – for example, relationships, work, finances, legal or health?
- Does anyone frequently complain about your drinking?

If you have answered 'yes' to two or more of these questions, I'm afraid you have a serious addiction problem. It is advisable that you request a medical examination to check on your health situation. People in the early stages of alcohol addiction are likely to have not yet developed serious health problems. It certainly won't be helping their gout, however.

Accepting that alcohol is a problem in your life has to be your first important step towards recovery. If you have tried and failed to overcome the addiction in the past, give yourself another chance. You don't have to tackle the problem alone – there are several responsible organizations that help people to defeat their alcoholism. (See the useful addresses at the back of this book for more information.)

Fluids

To reduce the risk of uric acid crystallizing in the joints (the cause of the severe pain in acute gout) it is important to drink plenty of fluids, obviously not including alcohol. Drinking a lot of fluids can also prevent uric acid crystals from being secreted into the urinary system as stones (known as *calculi*).

Besides water, it is fine to drink fluids such as fruit juices and herbal teas. However, as caffeine can stress adrenal glands that are overworked in any case where disease is present, it should be consumed in moderation, if at all.

A problem for many is finding an acceptable alternative to caffeine. Coffee, tea, cocoa and cola drinks can be replaced by fruit and vegetable juices and herbal teas – green tea is very good, as is rooibosch (redbush) tea.

If you are trying to lose weight, bear in mind that many soft drinks contain large amounts of sugar and should be avoided.

4

Eating to combat gout

The best means of treating gout naturally is via diet and nutrition, as discussed in this chapter. Being overweight appears to be the most common determining factor for excess uric acid production. Not all people with raised levels of uric acid, and ultimately gout, are overweight – as we have seen, kidney disease or genetic predisposition are two other causes of overproduction. However, it can safely be stated that the majority of gout sufferers are overweight to some degree, as several recent studies have shown. Losing weight should, therefore, be a priority – but avoid crash dieting as it can be counter-productive, increasing uric acid levels and causing an acute attack. Ideally, you should aim to lose no more than two pounds a week.

When a person with gout begins to lose weight, they are, for the following reasons, mounting a two-pronged attack on the cause of their disorder:

- The kidneys are more able to eliminate uric acid.
- In some cases, the production of uric acid by the liver is reduced.

Weight loss can also have the happy effect of moderating blood pressure. Obviously the risk of developing the disorders that high blood pressure can lead to is then much reduced.

How can I lose weight?

Starving yourself is not recommended as a means of parting with the pounds; neither is fad dieting where entire nutritional components are cut out, such as a carbohydrate-restricted diet, the 'cabbage-soup diet' and so on. It is important to choose a diet that is sustainable, which means eating a wide variety of healthy foods. Happily, changing to healthy eating will naturally cause weight loss in gout sufferers who are overweight; it will reduce levels of lipids (fats) in the blood; and it can reduce raised blood pressure.

However, it is essential that you *slowly* retrain your palate to accept different tastes. For this reason, it is advisable to cut back gradually on the amounts of sugar, salt and saturated fat you consume. It takes only 28 days of eating a food regularly for it to become a habit.

Keeping a diary

Keeping a food-intake diary is an excellent way of monitoring your progress. I suggest that you buy a notebook and devote a page to each day, listing all the foods you eat – including snacks and drinks.

Goals

It's a good idea to set goals on the very first page. For example, you may wish to make a goal of eating two types of vegetables each day. Without the diary, you may assume you have done badly – but upon reading your entries you may see that you've actually eaten two types of vegetables three or four times a week. That's a good starting point. Now you can focus on slowly increasing that amount.

As time goes by and you begin to achieve your goals as a matter of habit, list a new set of slightly more difficult ones.

Examples of long-term, general healthy eating goals are as follows:

● to eat two or three types of vegetables every day;
● to eat two or three portions of fruit every day;

- to eat nuts, seeds and dried fruit as snacks once or twice a day;
- to drink as much as 3.5 litres (6 pints) of water a day, including that in fruit and vegetable juices and green tea;
- to use vegetable oil, flower oil, corn oil or olive oil in cooking and dressing (extra virgin olive oil is best, and hemp oil, which is very nutritious, is also great for dressings);
- to minimize the amount of salt added to cooking and baking, and to avoid sprinkling it on food at the table;
- to reduce your intake of meat and dairy products, making sure to spread butter very thinly;
- to cut down on caffeine – coffee, chocolate, cola drinks, tea and cocoa;
- to cut down on alcohol (seek your doctor's advice if cutting down is a problem);
- to cut down on saturated fats;
- to cut down on table sugar and other sugar-containing products, such as cakes, sweets, biscuits and sugar-coated cereals;
- to cut out junk food;
- to cut out artificial sweeteners;
- to cut out fried foods (but see p. 49).

The reasons why many of the above foods should be minimized or cut out are explained later in this chapter. I will just add that if you are ultimately unable to eliminate certain foods, don't be discouraged. Reducing your intake should have a positive effect on your weight and the levels of uric acid in your blood. Ask your doctor to check your levels after changing your eating habits for a month or so – an indication that there is already less uric acid in your blood may give you an added incentive to persevere with your diet.

Help with cutting down

Changing the habits of a lifetime may be the hardest thing you have ever done, but for the sake of your health it is worth the effort. The following pointers may help you on your way:

- Eat one biscuit instead of two and cut yourself a smaller slice of cake prior to more drastically minimizing, or eliminating, foods containing sugar. If you find you are craving sugar, remember that the lift it offers will be brief – the next effect being a plummet into a low mood. Staving off hunger with fruit (fresh and dried), nuts and seeds is not only a far healthier choice, it also stabilizes blood-sugar levels, helping to ward off the low mood.
- Reduce your intake of caffeine products very gradually. Withdrawing too fast may cause fatigue and headaches.
- When drinking socially, order half pints of beer instead of pints, or drink alcohol-free wine, beers and lagers. Remember, it should not be necessary to eliminate alcohol entirely, unless you have an addiction to it, of course. In this event, you would be best advised to enlist the help of your doctor or a local Alcoholics Anonymous group.
- Stock fresh foods.
- Get into the habit of snacking on a variety of nuts, such as almonds, cashews, walnuts, Brazils and pecans; dried fruit, such as raisins, dates and apricots; and even seeds, such as pumpkin, hemp, sesame and sunflower. These should not spoil your appetite for an upcoming meal. Obviously, if you suffer from a nut allergy, leave nuts alone.
- Select a salad instead of fries when eating out.
- Slowly increase the number and variety of fruits and vegetables you use.
- Gradually reduce the amount of salt you add to your food and in cooking, especially if high blood pressure is already a problem. Remember that salt is commonly used as a

preservative and added to most processed, pre-packaged foods. Rock salt and sea salt are healthier alternatives, but should still be used sparingly.

- Eat three or four small meals a day, with some snacks in between.
- Never go more than two to three hours without eating – which means you should never go hungry. This will help control your blood-sugar levels.
- Don't skip breakfast. After fasting during the night, the body requires the glucose obtained from foods. Studies have shown that when a meal is missed, brain function can be compromised.
- Avoid missing other meals. When we allow ourselves to become very hungry, the sugary, high-fat foods that are bad for us become more tempting.
- Listen to your body. Stop eating when you feel satiated.
- Overeating creates a large mass of undigested food, and many associated problems.
- Don't mistake thirst for hunger. As the body's thirst mechanism is poorly developed, determine whether you really are hungry and don't simply need a drink.
- Don't use your stomach as an emotional rubbish bin. Try to find other outlets for your feelings, such as yoga, pilates and t'ai chi.
- Relax for at least ten minutes before starting each meal. Don't rush off straight after eating.
- Eat unhurriedly and chew thoroughly. Enjoy your food.
- At least half of your calorie intake should be made up of complex carbohydrates (see p. 53). These include fruits, vegetables and grains such as couscous and brown rice.
- Fats (oils) should be an important part of your diet. *Unsaturated* fats (also known as polyunsaturated fats) are greatly beneficial to health. These include olive, safflower, sunflower and corn oils. *Saturated* fats are largely derived from animals

and should be consumed in moderation, if at all. Examples are lard, suet, butter and dripping.

- If you are trying to reduce your intake of purines, remember to replace them with sufficient protein foods.
- Eat plenty of fibre in the form of fruits, vegetables, breads, cereals and legumes (not dried peas and beans).
- Try not to shop when you feel hungry. You won't then be so tempted to buy the less healthy foods.
- Drink as much water as possible, particularly during a flare-up of gout.
- Try to exercise regularly. You can lose weight more success- fully when you exercise and cut down food intake.
- Try to avoid stress. Gout is often triggered during or after a particularly stressful time.

So exactly what foods should I eat?

Dr John McDougall, a prominent promoter of hygienist and naturopath health principles, recommends that his gout patients follow a low-fat diet with no animal products whatsoever. He also advises that they eliminate highly allergenic plant foods such as wheat, corn and citrus fruits, claiming that benefits will be seen within a few days. He believes that the things we eat can cause arthritic disease by contributing to the formation of 'complexes' within the immune system – complexes acting much like slivers of wood stuck under the skin, causing severe inflammation of the joints.[4] Most doctors are of a less radical persuasion, however, recommending that their patients cut down on purine foods and monitor the effects. It is only when gout flare-ups persist regardless of your efforts that you should maybe try to cut out animal products altogether and, if that fails, cut out wheat, corn and citrus fruits, as Dr McDougall rec- ommends – these plant foods are widely recognized as having allergenic properties and being of some detriment to people with arthritic disease. Of course, if you would prefer to follow his recommendations at the outset, good for you. You should soon know whether your diet was the problem.

From the previous chapter you may now have an idea that you should eat lots of fruit, vegetables, grains and nuts. The following short sections should clarify the foods you would be best advised to cut down on and those that are better for you. I will just add that the World Health Organization recommends that we each consume five portions of fruit and five portions of vegetables a day. As ten portions is a lot for most people to achieve, I suggest that you try to eat a total of at least five portions a day in some combination of fruit and vegetables. Each of the following is equivalent to one portion:

- 100 g (3½ oz) of a very large fruit such as melon or pineapple
- one large fruit such as orange, banana or apple
- two medium fruits, such as kiwi fruits, plums or satsumas
- 100 ml (3½ fl oz) freshly squeezed fruit or vegetable juice
- 100 g (3½ oz) berries or cherries
- a large bowl of salad
- 90 g (3 oz), cooked weight, green vegetables
- 80 g (2¾ oz), cooked weight, root vegetables such as carrot or swede – don't include potatoes, sweet potatoes or yams
- 70 g (2½ oz), cooked weight, small vegetables such as peas or sweetcorn
- 80 g (2¾ oz) pulses, such as lentils.

Reducing sugar and refined carbohydrates

In his research, Professor John Yudkin observed that people with gout eat far more sugar than others. He then discovered that sugar actually increases the amount of uric acid in the blood, which gives us yet another cause of the development of gout. Unfortunately, our diets today are often high in sugar and refined carbohydrates, such as biscuits, cakes and pastries. Sugar contains no nutritional value at all. In fact, sugar consumption has been linked with many disorders, from diabetes to heart disease and cancer. You probably know that sugar converts into energy. What you may not know is that we can actually obtain all the sugars and energy we need from fruit and complex (unrefined) carbohydrates, such as grains and lentils, which convert into sugar in the body as nature intended.

Reducing salt

Salt is commonly used as a preservative and added to most processed, pre-packaged foods – cornflakes, for example, are high in salt. As a result, people who eat a lot of processed foods may be consuming more salt than they realize, especially when that used in cooking and at the table is taken into account. Try using herbs and spices for flavouring, but in moderation. Sea salt contains more minerals than ordinary salt, but it is still salt – so use sparingly.

Reducing meat and dairy produce

It is only people who eat large amounts of purines who should try to reduce their purine intake. Red meat, particularly offal, and shellfish contain perhaps the highest levels. You should, therefore, try to eat a piece of offal meat weighing about 85 g (3 oz), or the size of the palm of your hand, no more than twice a week.

If you then suffer a flare-up of gout, it would obviously be best to cut out offal and shellfish completely. Poultry and fish are good sources of protein and oils, but they do contain purines. Limit your consumption of the fish high in purines, such as herring, sardines, scallops, mackerel, roe, shrimp, mussels and anchovies, and eat poultry no more than twice a week. If, after doing this, you continue to suffer attacks of gout, you would be well advised to eliminate all meats, poultry and fish from your diet, replacing them with other forms of protein, such as tofu, tempeh and miso.

Meat and dairy products contain arachidonic acid, a fatty acid that contributes to the inflammation experienced in arthritic conditions. In one study,[5] arthritis sufferers reported a complete absence of symptoms after following a fat-free diet for seven weeks. Interestingly, when fats were reintroduced into their diets their symptoms returned. It is recommended, therefore, that people with gout cut down on the amount of meat and dairy produce they eat, whether purine intake appears to be the cause of their hyperuricemia or not.

Reducing the wrong sort of fats

Fats (fatty acids) are the most concentrated sources of energy in our diet, one gram of fat providing the body with nine calories of energy. However, as you may be aware, some fats are beneficial to health, while others are capable of raising cholesterol levels. They can also cause a condition called hypertriglyceridemia, which is a causal factor in gout.

Fats can be categorized as follows:

- *Saturated fat* Believed to be implicated in the development of heart disease, saturated fat comes mainly from animal sources and is generally solid at room temperature. Although margarine was, for many years, believed to be a healthier choice over butter, nutritionists have now revised their opinion, for some of the fats in the margarine hydrogenation process are changed into trans-fatty acids, which the body metabolizes as if they were saturated fatty acids – the same as butter. Butter is a valuable source of oils and vitamin A, but should be used sparingly. Margarine, on the other hand, is an artificial product containing many additives.
- *Unsaturated fat* Unsaturated fat, including polyunsaturated fat and monounsaturated fat, has a protective effect on the heart and other organs. Omega 3 and omega 6 oils occur naturally in oily fish, nuts and seeds, and are usually liquid at room

temperature. Because there is recent evidence that a relative increase in consumption of unsaturated fats from nuts and oils can help to lower levels of uric acid, even with a relatively high intake of protein, it is recommended that people with gout use cold-pressed oil (olive, rapeseed, hempseed, safflower and sunflower oil) daily, for dressings and in cooking. Extra virgin olive oil is best suited to cooking, however, as it suffers less damage from heat than other oils.

I must add that the process of frying changes the molecular structure of foods, rendering them potentially damaging to the body. If you must fry something, it is best to use a small amount of extra virgin olive oil and to cook at a low temperature. A healthier alternative is to sauté in a little water or tomato juice, or to grill, bake and steam. Stir-frying is good – but by this I mean cooking the food in a little *water* and just drizzling on olive oil afterwards. If you love chips, coat thick fingers of potato with olive oil before baking in the oven. They're not only healthier this way, they taste better too!

Omega 3 versus omega 6 fatty acids

Although I mentioned above that essential fatty acids (EFAs) are important for reducing inflammation, I would like to explain the value of a good dietary balance between omega 3 and omega 6 EFAs. Both of these EFAs are beneficial to health – but it's not that simple. The two are metabolically different and have opposing physiological functions. Both are of benefit in different ways, but only if your diet is balanced approximately 2:1 in favour of omega 3. In other words, double the intake of omega 3 over omega 6 is required for optimum benefit. Research has indicated that individuals with this balance appear to be less likely to have heart disease, hypertension, arthritis, cancer, other inflammatory disease and autoimmune disorders. On the other hand, people who consume more omega 6 than 3 are likely to have an increased incidence of cardiovascular disease and inflammatory disorders.

Unfortunately, the modern diet has an excess of omega 6 and a shortfall of omega 3, which can cause or worsen inflammation and circulatory problems. I was actually quite shocked to learn that, in general, most people consume between 10 and 20 times more omega 6 than omega 3! As getting the balance of these EFAs is so very important, it can be assumed that the majority of the population in the West need to eat more omega 3 and cut back on the amount of omega 6 they consume. You don't need to bring your calculator into the kitchen either, you just need to concentrate on including more omega 3 EFAs in your diet.

The top food sources of omega 3 EFAs include fish and seafood (such as fresh tuna, sardines, halibut, shrimp, snapper, cod, salmon and scallops), as well as flax seed, walnuts, winter squash, olive oil, soy beans, kidney beans and tofu. Flax seeds and walnuts have the highest omega 3 content of all. They can be sprinkled on to salads, baked potatoes, porridge, muesli and granola.

Omega 3 is now increasingly being added to everyday foods by companies who are cashing in on the media hype, and for once we can be thankful of this. These foods include certain types of bread, yoghurt, fruit juice, baked beans and tinned pasta. Look at the list of ingredients.

Eggs

Contrary to long-held opinion, the cholesterol in eggs is not now thought to be a risk factor for health. Eggs contain lecithin, a superb biological detergent capable of breaking down fats so that they can be utilized by the body. In addition, lecithin prevents the accumulation of too many acid or alkaline substances in the blood and encourages the transport of nutrients through the cell walls. Buy free-range eggs and eat them soft-boiled or poached, as a hard yolk will bind the lecithin, rendering it useless as a fat-detergent.

The Food Standards Agency now states that most people don't need to limit their consumption of eggs so long as they are part of a balanced diet.

Fresh fruit and vegetables

Try to eat five portions of fruit and vegetables on a daily basis – but only small amounts of asparagus, mushrooms and cauliflower, which are high in purines. Make a variety of salads and try to eat one every day. When you cook vegetables, boil them in the minimum of unsalted (or lightly salted) water for the minimum amount of time. Lightly steaming or stir-frying (as above) are healthy alternatives.

Legumes (peas and beans)

Because all peas and beans contain moderate amounts of purines, try to limit the amount you eat. The soya bean and soya products, such as soya milk, tofu, tempeh and miso, also contain purines (see p. 52), so should also be eaten in moderation.

Nuts

Nuts, on the other hand, should be an intrinsic part of your diet. All nuts contain vital nutrients, but almonds, cashews, Brazils and pecans perhaps offer the greatest array. Eat a wide assortment as snacks, with cereals and in baking.

Grains

Wheat is our staple grain in the West, refined wheat flour the product with which most of our cakes, pastries, biscuits and breads are made. However, wheat (and corn, to a lesser extent) is known to be particularly acid-forming, and people with gout would be well advised to limit the amount of wheat products they eat. More beneficial grains are oats, barley, bran, brown rice, couscous, millet, rye, spelt and quinoa. These are all excellent sources of protein, complex carbohydrates (see p. 54), fibre, vitamins and minerals. Try eating rice cakes, oatmeal biscuits and cake, carob cake, scones (made with ground rice) and carrot cake (made with brown-rice flour).

Now that we have established what foods we ought to be eating, it's time to think about how we might combine them, in the right proportions, to arrive at a healthily balanced diet geared to gout. Depending on how active you are, you should be eating in total between 1,800 and 3,000 calories a day. The following sections should help you achieve that intake in the right balance. I also offer advice on food combining and supplements, followed by suggested menus to get you started.

Protein

Many protein foods are high in purines, which we know are a problem in gout. Many experts recommend, therefore, that the intake of protein should not exceed 25 per cent of your total calorie intake per day. I know it is difficult to judge the exact amount of a particular food in your diet. However, if you at least try to consume the recommended amounts of meat, as well as fruit, vegetables, nuts, seeds, legumes, soft-boiled egg yolks, soya products and so on, you will be in the right region. Remember, too, that you can lower your levels of uric acid even if you are not able to follow this diet to the letter. Try to do the best you can and appreciate the fact that you are helping your body to fight this disease.

One study into the value of reducing protein in gout has suggested that eating tofu, which is made from the soya bean and is a source of complete protein, is a better choice than meats. However, soya products do contain purines, albeit in lesser amounts than meat, so should not be consumed every day. There are many soya bean products, including soya milk, tofu, tempeh and miso. Tofu is particularly versatile and can be used in both savoury and sweet dishes (see the further reading section for details of an excellent tofu cookbook).

If you find that you are eating considerably less than the recommended amount of protein, I strongly advise that you take free-form amino acids, which are available from healthfood shops. The herb acidophilus is also useful, taken twice a day.

Recommended protein consumption

The following measurements should give you a rough idea not only of your protein intake, but also of your total calorific consumption (examples of carbohydrate and fat calories are given later in this chapter). Use them in conjunction with the recommended proportion of protein intake within total calorie intake that was noted above (25 per cent).

Here are the calorific values of some common protein foods:

- 28 g (1 oz) grilled haddock – a very small piece – yields 40 calories;
- 28 g (1 oz) roasted chicken – also a very small piece – yields 40 calories;
- 28 g (1 oz) cottage cheese yields 15 calories;
- 28 g (1 oz) Parmesan cheese yields 120 calories;
- 28 g (1 oz) soya bean yields 50 calories.

Butter, which contains some protein, is very high in fat – 28 g (1 oz) of butter contains 226 calories. I reiterate, therefore, that butter should be used very sparingly.

Carbohydrates

Our digestive systems break down carbohydrates into simple sugars that are used to fuel essential body processes such as brain function, nervous system function and muscle activity. In short, we obtain vital energy from carbohydrate-containing foods. A word of warning, however: any excess carbohydrate is converted to fat by insulin, the 'fat-storage' hormone.

To ensure that fats and proteins are effectively broken down, and to guarantee the production of sufficient energy, we need to eat plenty of what are known as complex carbohydrates. These include fruit, vegetables and grains (breads, pasta, brown rice, cereals, couscous, millet, barley, bulgar wheat and other cereals). On the other hand, so-called simple carbohydrates will only pile on the pounds and cause levels of uric acid to rise. They include table sugar and the sugars found in sweets, cakes, biscuits and sweetened cereals. The sugar in these foods causes erratic fluctuations in blood-sugar levels – meaning that after consuming them you will experience a spurt of energy, followed by a dip into a low mood. Here we have yet another reason why simple carbohydrates should be avoided as much as possible. Try to snack on a variety of fruit and nuts instead of cakes and biscuits. If you are persistent, you should soon lose that urge for sweet foods.

Recommended carbohydrate consumption

Remember that we should all try to eat at least five portions of fruit and vegetables a day. We can go some way towards meeting that target just by eating enough of the right sort of carbohydrates. For people with gout it is recommended that 55 per cent of their daily calorific intake be in the form of carbohydrate. If you are trying to lose weight, here are the calorific values of some recommended sources of complex carbohydrates:

- 28 g (1 oz) banana yields 22 calories;
- 28 g (1 oz) orange yields 12 calories;
- 28 g (1oz) apple yields 17 calories;
- 28 g (1 oz) wholemeal pasta yields 35 calories;
- 28 g (1 oz) wholemeal bread yields 38 calories;
- 28 g (1 oz) cabbage yields 4 calories.

Do bear in mind that wholemeal foods are moderately high in purines and have allergenic properties (see pp. 35 and 51), and should therefore be eaten in moderation.

Fats and oils

As already noted, fats (fatty acids) are the most concentrated sources of energy in our diet. Foods containing good (unsaturated) fat – omega 3 and omega 6 – are crucial to good health (see pp. 48–50). Oils are also a natural source of vitamin E, which is an important antioxidant. (Antioxidants mop up damaging 'free radicals' that build up in the cells of the body and are part of any disease process.) However, remember that saturated fat, when consumed regularly, can lead to the development of heart disease. Eating fried foods is not recommended for people with gout – grill your food instead.

Recommended unsaturated fat consumption

It is estimated that most adults consume approximately 42 per cent of their total daily calories as fat – most of it saturated. However, the recommended daily intake is 20 per cent. Eating the necessary unsaturated fats will ensure reduced calorie intake and greater energy provision. It will also reduce the risk of developing hypertriglyceridemia (see Chapter 1).

Here are the calorific values of some fat-containing foods:

- 28 g (1 oz) oil yields 130 calories;
- 28 g (1 oz) butter yields 226 calories;
- 28 g (1 oz) egg yields 80 calories;
- 28 g (1 oz) oily fish yields 60 calories.

Fibre (roughage)

Fibre, formerly known as roughage, is the indigestible part of plants. It is the cellulose fibres forming the leaf webbing in green vegetables, the skins of sweetcorn and beans, and the husks of wheat and corn. Fibre – a type of carbohydrate – is found in fruits, vegetables, nuts, seeds, beans, peas, lentils, wholemeal breads and cereals (wheat, oats, rye, barley, quinoa, spelt, buckwheat, corn and so on).

It is estimated that people in the West consume only 12 g (under ½ oz) of fibre on average per day, instead of the recommended 20–30 g (about 1 oz). However, the latter amount was, in fact, consumed up to the time of the Second World War. Fibre is useful not only because of its high nutritional value, but also because it is a bulking agent that quickly sweeps the bowel clean, ensuring no unhealthy waste products lurk in hidden corners.

When waste products persistently linger in the bowel, as occurs in low-fibre diets, toxins are absorbed back into the bloodstream causing eventual weakening of the immune system. The slower and more regulated absorption of glucose into the bloodstream is also aided by fibre – as a consequence of which the individual avoids plummeting into hunger troughs and craving sugar to raise blood-sugar levels. Another advantage of fibre is that the appetite is satiated on comparatively fewer calories. All in all, fibre is an essential food component and crucial to improved health.

The only form of fibre you may wish to cut down on is wheat. This cereal is a common allergen (see p. 45), and because it is acid-forming it can contribute to raised levels of uric acid in the blood.

Food combining

Many foods are not easily digested when eaten together. The Hay system of food combining recommends, for example, that high-protein foods (such as meats, dairy produce, eggs, fish, nuts and soya) should not be eaten at the same meal as high-carbohydrate foods (such as rice, potatoes and bread) because proteins require an acid medium in the stomach to be broken down whereas carbohydrates require an alkaline medium. This means that the bulk of the diet should be fruits, salad and vegetables, as these are not high in either carbohydrate or protein.

Some people with arthritic disease, including gout, have claimed to feel much better within a few days of commencing a food combining diet. (For details of the Hay system of food combining, see the useful addresses section.)

Food supplements

When an individual is in a state of dis-ease, their nutritional requirements are increased for various reasons. There is thus a strong case for taking good quality food supplements in a sensible manner. Steer clear of vitamin A supplementation as it is believed to increase the risk for gout attacks. Also, as you will read below, garlic and vitamin C (the latter in large quantities) – which were formerly thought to be of benefit in gout – are now known to cause more harm than good.

The following supplements are recommended in gout:

Pantothenic acid and vitamin B complex

In order to excrete uric acid, the body needs sufficient of the B vitamins, particularly pantothenic acid – also known as vitamin B5. This vitamin is crucial for the production of the anti-stress hormones, the release of energy from protein, carbohydrates, fats and sugars, and for good health of the nervous system. It is interesting to note that gout often follows times of stress, and stress depletes the body of the B vitamins. This may be the reason why gout sufferers are typically deficient in the B vitamins and why supplementation can be useful.

The suggested dosage of pantothenic acid for gout treatment is 500 mg twice daily, one dose taken with breakfast and one with the evening meal. Follow the label dosage instructions for the B complex vitamins.

Vitamin C

One of the more potent antioxidants, vitamin C is the main anti-stress vitamin, and is probably the most important nutrient for immune system function. One study[6] found that when vitamin C was added to the diet of elderly people with arthritis and gout, pain levels were significantly reduced. This is probably because vitamin C is a powerful *urosoric* agent, meaning that it assists the kidneys in eliminating uric acid. Indeed, it works in much the same way as the medication *probenecid.*

Be careful not to consume very large amounts of vitamin C, however, as this causes uric acid to crystallize in the kidneys, increasing the risk of uric acid-based kidney stones.

Garlic (Allium sativum)

Garlic has been recommended since the very earliest of times for the prevention and treatment of gout. There is no doubt that garlic can ward off infection and help fight cancer and heart disease – however, I can find no evidence that it lowers uric acid levels or reduces inflammation and pain. Moreover, it is now known to block blood-clotting agents in the body, meaning that an injury can causing profuse bleeding that may be difficult to stem. Experts are actually now asserting that garlic can be dangerous when taken with non-steroidal anti-inflammatory drugs (NSAIDs). This is because peptic ulcers can arise and when these burst this may result in a life-threatening bleed.

For all these reasons, I have to recommend that a person with gout eats only small amounts of garlic, and completely avoids garlic supplements.

Cod liver oil

Recent research has strongly suggested that the age-old belief that cod liver oil is good for the joints is true. A study in Cardiff[6] found that cod liver oil might delay or even reverse the destruction of joint cartilage and inflammatory pain associated with joint disease. Make sure that you purchase the variety containing EPA and DHA – fish oil concentrates – since it is probably more effective. Follow the instructions on the label.

Burdock root

Research has shown that burdock root is a fairly powerful xanthine oxidase inhibitor – xanthine oxidase being an enzyme in the body that produces uric acid. Medications such as allopurinol actually work by blocking this enzyme. As burdock root is a natural treatment, it can be used in conjunction with prescription medications. You may even wish to speak to your doctor about the possibility of trying out burdock root before you commit yourself to taking a long-term drug.

Unfortunately, burdock root is also a diuretic (it causes the body to lose fluids), so you need to keep well hydrated while taking it. It is available in tablet form or as dried root that can be brewed up into a tea.

Celery seed

Celery seed has been used as an alternative treatment for gout for over two thousand years. I could find no evidence that it lowers uric acid levels or reduces inflammation and pain, however. It is also a diuretic, which means that your levels of uric acid will increase if insufficient fluids are drunk while you are taking it. All in all, I wouldn't advise that you use this particular herb.

Glucosamine and chondroitin

Although many people with arthritic pain (including gout) take glucosamine and chondroitin on a daily basis, recent studies showed no improvement at all in volunteer patients. Therefore it was concluded that these supplements are no more effective than a placebo (simple sugar pill) in relieving symptoms. Glucosamine is not recommended for use within the NHS.

MSM (organic sulphur)

Although there is no evidence to prove its efficacy, MSM (extracted from tree bark) has become one of the best-selling herbal remedies for the treatment of arthritic conditions. It is actually an organic sulphur which is said to replace the natural sulphurs that are so easily destroyed in the food we eat.

Many companies supply petrochemical MSM. However, try to ensure that your purchase is petrochemical-free. (For details of a supplier of petrochemical-free MSM, see the useful addresses section.) MSM is available in tablet form, vegetarian capsules or powder to blend with food or drinks. The suggested dosage is 1–6 g a day.

Examination of some popular remedies

In this section I look at whether or not some popular remedies seem to do what they are supposed to do.

Noni juice

Noni juice is derived from the fruit of the *Morinda citrifolia* tree, which commonly flourishes in Polynesia. The pungent odour of the fruit when ripening has earned it the informal name of 'cheese fruit' or 'vomit fruit'. The pulp, bark, leaves and seeds of the noni fruit have been used as a healing tonic for inflammation, constipation, respiratory problems and so on for over two thousand years. In recent years, the bitter-tasting juice of the fruit has been mixed with more palatable fruit flavours and marketed in the West as 'a miracle in a bottle'. As a consequence, the manufacture of noni juice is a multi-million dollar industry with a loyal following; many swear by its health benefits, although there are apparently wide inconsistencies in patient testimonials. It is actually said that the Polynesians themselves only resort to using the juice as a health tonic when all other avenues have failed.

There is no doubt that noni fruit powder is rich in carbohydrates, fibre and other beneficial health-giving agents. However, when the juice of the noni fruit was analysed in laboratories in recent years, a surprisingly small quantity of these nutrients were detected. Indeed, one medicinal portion of noni juice was found to contain no more health-giving properties than are present in one orange. It was concluded, therefore, that the high nutrient content of noni is stored in the pulp of the fruit rather than in the juice.

In 1998, the manufacturers of noni juice were charged by the Attorneys General of several US states with making unfounded health claims. They were ordered to stop advertising the purported benefits until scientific back-up was provided. This has not happened and the juice continues to be advertised in other US states. In 2007, immunologist Dr Jeffrey Galpin reviewed the studies on noni juice and made it clear that the claims of manufacturers have not been backed up. 'It's promoted to do everything with no validation of anything,' he said.

France has warned prospective customers of the risks of noni juice, saying that severe liver problems were found in some people after consumption of the juice. It should therefore not be used by people with liver problems. Constipation is a common side effect of taking the juice, particularly if high amounts are consumed. A further possible side effect is coughing and wheezing. If you still wish to try noni juice, it is recommended that you visit your doctor before starting to take it. You should build up intake very gradually, monitoring the effect very carefully.

Aloe juice

The aloe vera plant has a long history as a folk remedy and is known all over the world as the 'first aid plant' or 'medicine plant'. Both the gel and the latex can be extracted from the plant, the gel being a clear, jelly-like pulp from the inner part of the leaves and the latex being a bitter yellow substance that is carried in tiny tubes beneath the outer skin of the leaves. It is the latex that is commonly known as 'aloe juice' and is now widely used to treat a variety of conditions including digestive tract problems, all types of arthritis and gout.

Experts claim that aloe juice is packed with a particular combination of nutrients that work together to relieve the pain of chronic conditions such as arthritis and gout. Aloe juice is also high in 'basic sugars' (known as *mucopolysaccharides*), which are normally present in every cell in the body and need replenishment on a regular basis. These substances, in combination, are believed to make aloe juice an immune system stimulant, a powerful anti-inflammatory and a good analgesic (painkiller). Whether or not this remedy can actually lower uric acid levels into the bargain is another question entirely – and I can find no evidence of research into this.

The fact that some experts are convinced that aloe juice can reduce inflammation and pain, prevent further damage and actually repair diseased tissue may make it worth a trial. It is said that the degree of success with aloe juice treatment varies considerably from person to person. I can only assume that this therapy is more successful if used in the early stages of a disease and perhaps in people who don't smoke and are making other positive lifestyle changes to improve their condition, as mentioned in this book. Aloe juice is composed of plant nutrients rather than the chemicals found in drugs. The side effects linked to aloe juice are rare, but in a small number of people it can apparently cause electrolyte loss, fluid imbalance, intestinal cramps and slow healing of wounds. However, these side effects should only arise if you take large doses for a prolonged period. If you follow the label instructions, side effects will not normally occur. Despite inadequate research into aloe juice and gout, it would appear that taking the substance can do no harm. Indeed, it may even be of benefit. This is another area in which further research would be welcome and we can only hope that this shortly takes place.

Apple cider vinegar

Apple cider vinegar is seen by many as a miraculous tonic containing a powerful combination of healing properties. People who advocate the use of this product claim that it contains dozens of beneficial components which have an anti-ageing effect, preventing germs, parasites and infectious diseases from invading the body and combating a variety of ailments such as chronic fatigue, diabetes, digestive problems and migraines. It is also claimed to help reduce high blood pressure and high cholesterol.

Perhaps apple cider vinegar is best known, however, as a curative for arthritic disease, inclusive of gout. Exponents of this substance believe that apple cider vinegar dissolves the harmful acid crystals so that they can be flushed from the body in the urine, effectively stopping the disease process and encouraging the body to heal itself. It must be said that there is no denying the bulk of anecdotal evidence from people with arthritis to support this belief. Indeed, many people with arthritis profess to have benefited greatly and plenty claim complete recovery as a result.

You may be interested to know, however, that there is now a growing body of experts who strongly oppose the notion that apple cider vinegar has medicinal properties. They state that there is absolutely no scientific evidence to back up the anecdotal claims and that apple cider vinegar is anything but a storehouse of nutrients. Taking one to two teaspoonfuls two to three times daily of the product (with honey) is recommended, yet when one teaspoonful was subjected to nutritional analysis less than one gram of carbohydrate and only minuscule amounts of calcium, iron, magnesium, sodium, manganese, potassium and phosphorus were found. Moreover, there was no fibre, no vitamins and no amino acids, contrary to claims by proponents of this therapy. Scientists believe that any beneficial enzymes would be unable to survive the acid environment of vinegar, and if they did, they would quickly be destroyed by stomach acid.

Although the arthritis associations I contacted declined to offer their opinions on apple cider vinegar, the Arthritis Foundation refers to it on their website as 'a harmless, but unproven, arthritis remedy'. It stresses that arthritis symptoms commonly come and go and that if an unproven remedy was used at a time when symptoms were in decline, it would be easy to think that the remedy had worked. The foundation states that this appears to be what has happened for plenty of people who use vinegar-related remedies.

Having said that, if you are taking apple cider vinegar and feel better for doing so, you should continue the regime. If something works for you, it works – whether or not the science backs it up. According to proponents of this regime, the best apple cider vinegar is ruddy in colour with a discernible amount of residue floating around in the bottle. One to three teaspoonfuls should be mixed into 8 fluid ounces of water three times daily and taken before meals. Honey can be mixed into the drink to make it more palatable.

Suggested menus

Note that the cup you should use for the measures given below is a small teacup or American cup measure rather than a mug. Any helpings of meat, poultry or fish should be no larger than the palm of your hand. Drinks are not included.

Day 1

Breakfast: 1 grapefruit followed by 2 slices of toast
Snack: ⅓ cup mixed sunflower seeds and almonds
Lunch: Salad with cottage cheese and chives
Snack: 1 cup cherries (if you are not already eating these every day)
Dinner: Irish stew with a very small amount of lean beef
Snack: 2 oatcakes

Day 2

Breakfast: Porridge with cracked linseed, honey and rice milk, 1 tofu yoghurt
Snack: 1 banana
Lunch: 2 soft-poached eggs on wholemeal toast, 1 potato scone
Snack: ⅓ cup pecan nuts
Dinner: Grilled chicken breast with potatoes, carrots and parsnips
Snack: ⅓ cup dried apricots

Day 3

Breakfast: 1 large wedge of canteloupe melon, 2 Ryvita wafers
Snack: 1 carob bar (available from healthfood shops)
Lunch: 1 large baked potato with tuna, 2 oatcakes
Snack: ⅓ cup mixed dried fruit and nuts
Dinner: Home-made chicken curry with brown rice, pear
Snack: 2 slices wholemeal toast with jam

Day 4
Breakfast: Muesli with low-fat milk and chopped banana
Snack: 2 oatcakes
Lunch: Tomato soup with roll, 1 yoghurt
Snack: ⅓ cup dried apricots
Dinner: Grilled wild salmon with potatoes, broccoli and carrots
Snack: 1 cup mixed fruit and nuts

Day 5
Breakfast: Porridge with cracked linseed, honey and soya milk, 2 Ryvita wafers
Snack: ⅓ cup pecan nuts
Lunch: 2 grilled kippers with grilled tomatoes and scrambled egg
Snack: 2 kiwi fruit
Dinner: Mixed vegetable casserole, rice pudding made with rice milk
Snack: 2 slices wholemeal toast

Day 6
Breakfast: Fresh fruit salad, soft-boiled egg with toast fingers
Snack: 2 oatcakes
Lunch: Baked potato with cottage cheese and pineapple, slice of carob cake
Snack: ⅓ cup mixed nuts
Dinner: Falafel (similar to a veggie burger and available from healthfood shops) with chips baked in the oven (see p. 49)
Snack: 1 orange

Day 7
Breakfast: 2 slices wholemeal toast with raw honey, banana
Snack: 2 rice cakes (available from healthfood shops)
Lunch: Mixed salad, baked apple

Snack:	Pear
Dinner:	Baked wild salmon with potatoes, broccoli and carrots
Snack:	1 slice carrot cake

You may wish to eat a bowlful of cherries every day, too, to help ward off gout attacks.

5

Complementary therapies

Complementary medicine has been described as all the therapies not taught in medical school. It includes such techniques as acupuncture, homeopathy and reflexology. You may know these as 'alternative therapies' – but this term can be misleading. The word alternative suggests that the therapy can be used to replace conventional medicine. Unfortunately, in treating gout this is rarely the case.

Complementary therapies are suitable for treating disease for the following reasons:

- they have non-invasive qualities;
- they are largely free from side effects;
- they can be used in addition to long-term medication;
- most of them are enjoyable.

People who use complementary therapies do report substantial benefits, although some of these may derive from simply knowing that they are doing something positive to help themselves. Different therapies appear to suit different people.

Acupressure

Acupressure is an ancient form of oriental healing, combining acupuncture and massage. Practitioners of this technique use the thumb, fingertip or the palm of the hand to firmly massage certain pressure points located at specific sites throughout the body. These points are the same as those used in acupuncture (see p. 69). Neither oils nor equipment are used in this type of therapy.

68

Acupressure is believed to enhance the body's own healing mechanisms. Pain relief is sometimes rapid. However, improvements can take longer in chronic conditions. At some hospitals in the UK, acupressure is available as part of the physiotherapy treatment options.

Acupuncture

Also an ancient form of oriental healing, acupuncture involves puncturing the skin with fine needles at specific points in the body. These points are located along energy channels (meridians) that are believed to correspond to certain internal organs. The energy itself is known as *chi*. Needles are inserted to increase, decrease or unblock the flow of chi energy so that the balance of yin and yang is restored. Yin, the female force, is calm and passive; it also represents dark, cold, swelling and moisture. On the other hand, yang, the male force, is stimulating and aggressive, representing heat, light, contraction and dryness. It is thought that an imbalance in these forces is the cause of illness and disease. For example, a person who feels the cold, and suffers fluid retention and fatigue, would be considered to have an excess of yin. A person suffering from headaches, however, will be deemed to have an excess of yang.

Emotional, physical or environmental factors are believed to disturb the chi energy balance, and can also be treated. For example, acupuncture has been used to alleviate stress, digestive disorders, insomnia, asthma and allergies. Studies have shown that treatment promotes the brain to release endorphins and encephalins (natural painkillers), boost the immune system and calm the nervous system. It can be seen, then, that acupuncture has many applications.

A qualified acupuncturist will use a set method to determine acupuncture points – it is thought that there are as many as 2,000 such points on the body. At a consultation, questions may be asked about lifestyle, sleeping patterns, fears, phobias and reactions to stress. The pulses will be felt, then the acupuncture itself carried out, fine needles being placed in the relevant sites. The first consultation will normally last an hour, and patients should feel improvements after four to six sessions.

In treating gout, this traditional Chinese medicine advocates that an over-rich diet causes a build-up of damp and heat internally, causing phlegm to stagnate and bringing about disturbance of the spleen and kidneys. Treatment, therefore, involves placing fine needles in the spleen and stomach acupuncture points. Other local points are used according to the joint affected by gout.

In one important study in China,[7] 54 volunteers with arthritis were given a form of acupuncture (warm needling in this case) in which the needles are dipped in Zhuifengsu, a Chinese herb. As a consequence, every volunteer reported a decrease in their pain. In another study, in Russia, into auriculo-electropuncture (AEP)[8] – treatment of acupuncture points on the ear – all 16 arthritis patients felt better after treatment, showing 'statistically significant' improvement in their blood samples. The results of these studies are believed to apply to all types of arthritis, including gout.

Acupuncture is now losing its unorthodox reputation, and has made much headway in the West. In recent years it has gained so much respect in the medical field that many doctors now perform the therapy.

Bioelectromagnetics

Bioelectromagnetics is the study of how living organisms – all of which produce electrical currents – interact with magnetic fields. The electrical currents within our bodies are capable of creating magnetic fields that extend outside our bodies, and these fields can be influenced by external magnetic forces. In fact, specific external magnetism can actually produce physical and behavioural changes. Just as drugs induce a response in their target tissues, so low magnetic fields can produce a chosen biological response – but without the chemical side effects associated with drugs.

External magnetism cannot only correct abnormalities in the energy fields of patients with disease, effectively working as a healer, it is also capable of stabilizing a chronic condition – although certainly not in every case. As a pain reliever, external magnetism is becoming ever more widely used, and much experimentation is currently under way. Electromagnetic apparatus is even becoming a regular fixture of NHS treatment rooms. This apparatus creates a pulsed magnetic field, which is used to aid the recovery of bone fractures, tendon and ligament tears and muscle injuries, for example. A small, light, comparatively inexpensive version can be purchased for easy-to-wear home use. External magnetism should not be used by anyone fitted with a heart pacemaker.

External magnetism in the form of a specially designed wrist appliance – worn like a wristwatch – is also believed to be effective in treating aches, pains and injuries in any region of the body. As with other types of external magnetism, this appliance is said to improve the ability of the blood to carry oxygen and nutrients around the body. It is also believed to speed the removal of toxins and other waste products. Various appliances are available for use on different parts of the body (see the useful addresses section for outlet details).

Homeopathy

The homeopathic approach to medicine is holistic, which means that the overall health of a person – physical, emotional and psychological – is assessed before treatment commences. Those who practise homeopathy believe that the whole make-up of a person determines the disorders to which he or she is prone, and their likely symptoms. After a thorough consultation, the homeopath will offer a remedy compatible with the patient's symptoms as well as with their temperament and characteristics. Consequently, two individuals with the same disorder may be offered entirely different remedies.

Homeopathic remedies are derived from plant, mineral and animal substances, which are soaked in alcohol to extract what are known as the 'live' ingredients. This initial solution is then diluted many times, being vigorously shaken each time to add energy. Impurities are removed and the remaining solution made up into tablets, ointments, powders or suppositories. Interestingly, low dilution remedies are used for severe symptoms while high dilution remedies are used for milder symptoms.

Since antiquity, the homeopathic concept has been that 'like cures like'. The full healing abilities of this type of remedy were first recognized in the early nineteenth century, when a German doctor, Samuel Hahnemann, noticed that the herbal cure for malaria – which was based on an extract of cinchona bark (quinine) – actually produced symptoms of malaria. Further tests convinced him that the production of mild symptoms caused the body to fight the disease. He went on to treat malaria patients successfully with dilute doses of cinchona bark.

Each homeopathic remedy is first 'proved' by being taken by a healthy person – usually a volunteer homeopath – and having the symptoms noted. This remedy is then known to be capable of curing the same symptoms in an ill person. The whole idea of proving and using homeopathic remedies can be difficult to comprehend as it is exactly the opposite to how conventional medicines operate. For example, a patient who has a cold with a runny nose would be treated with a homeopathic remedy that would produce a runny nose in a healthy patient. Conventional medicine, on the other hand, would provide something that blocks up the nose.

Nowadays, a homeopathic remedy can be formulated to aid virtually every disorder. Although remedies are safe and non-addictive, occasionally the patient's symptoms may briefly worsen. This is known as a healing crisis and is usually short-lived. It is actually a good indication that the remedy is working well.

You should visit a homeopath if you have a medical problem that is not getting better or if you are continually swapping one set of symptoms for another. It is a common misconception that you can just pop along to your local chemist, look up your particular complaint on the homeopathic remedy chart and begin taking the remedy. If only it were that simple: homeopathic training takes several years, and a lot of knowledge and experience is required before practitioners can decide the correct remedies for complaints other than the very superficial. And as I mentioned earlier, what works for one person is not liable to work for another.

Selecting an appropriate remedy is only part of the procedure, however. The homeopath will also evaluate patient reaction to ascertain what, if any, further treatment is necessary.

Hydrotherapy (1)

In 400 BC, Hippocrates alleged that bathing was useful for a variety of conditions, and he included gout in his list. A long soak in a hot bath is profoundly relaxing. It also has a calming effect on the central nervous system. Even more soothing, sur-prisingly, is a long soak in a bath as close as possible to body temperature (37° C). For best results, the bathwater should cover your shoulders – and the longer you are immersed, the better you will feel. For comfort, place a folded towel beneath your head – although the water should provide adequate support as a body in water weighs only a quarter of its normal weight. Keep the temperature of the water as constant as possible by regularly topping up from the hot tap.

You may be interested to know that heart size increases by 30 per cent within six seconds of immersion in warm water, cardiac output increases by 34 per cent, blood pressure remains steady and changes within the sympathetic nervous system mean that there is a decreased perception of pain.

Hydrotherapy (2)

It is important for a person with gout to drink plenty of fluids. This reduces the risk of uric acid crystallizing in the joints (the cause of the severe pain in acute gout). Ideally, you should try to drink as much as 3.5 litres (6 pints) of water a day. It is fine to include other fluids in this amount, such as fruit juices and herbal teas. Try topping up fruit juices with water and keep a glass at your work station or in the kitchen so you can keep taking sips. If you can't manage to drink the recommended amount, don't worry – just drink as much as you can.

Hypnotherapy

Hypnotherapy may be described as psychotherapy using hypnosis. There is, however, still no acceptable definition for the actual state of hypnosis. It is commonly described as an altered state of consciousness, lying somewhere between being awake and asleep. People under hypnosis are aware of their surroundings, yet their minds are, to a large extent, under the control of the hypnotist. People under hypnosis also seem to pass control of their actions, as well as a chunk of their thoughts, to the hypnotist. We have all seen people under hypnosis on TV, acting out a role. At the time they are absorbed in what they have been told to do – often instigated by a specific trigger word – but immediately afterwards they wonder what on earth they were doing. Their behaviour had been dictated, to a certain degree, by the hypnotist. Hypnotherapy is about the hypnotist using this power for therapeutic purposes, and it is performed by the therapist putting the patient into a trance.

By the early nineteenth century, some physicians were using hypnotism – then called mesmerism – to perform pain-free operations. The majority of medical professionals were highly sceptical, however, believing that the patients had been either schooled – or paid – to show no pain. Not until the last two decades has hypnotism become an accepted form of therapy.

Nowadays, a hypnotherapist will take a full psychological and physiological history of each patient, and then will slowly talk the patient into a trance state. The therapist can either use direct suggestion – by indicating that the patient's pain, for example, will notably lessen – or will begin to explore the root cause of any tension, anxiety or depression.

Hypnotherapists have found that when, in chronic pain conditions, the level of tension is lowered, many of the physical symptoms are also greatly reduced. Some experts in the field believe that the main purpose of hypnotherapy is to aid relaxation, reduce tension and increase confidence and the ability to cope with problems. However, there has been at least one study into the effects of hypnotherapy on arthritic conditions. In this instance,[9] levels of beta endorphin, epinephrine, norepinephrine, dopamine and serotonin were measured in 19 patients before and after hypnosis. Following the therapy there were clinically and statistically significant decreases in pain, anxiety and depression, and increases in the endorphins that have a beneficial effect on the immune system. The conclusion was that hypnotherapy could well play an important role in conquering arthritic conditions, including gout.

One common fear is that the therapist may, while the patient is in a trance, implant dangerous suggestions or extract improper personal information. I can only say that patients can come out of a trance at any time – particularly if they are asked to do or say anything they would not even contemplate when awake. And malpractice would only have to be brought to light once to ruin the therapist's career. You may prefer to visit a hypnotherapist recommended by your doctor.

Relaxation and meditation

You may wonder how relaxation techniques and meditation can help a person with gout. Well, any activity that increases energy demands also increases the metabolism, which then produces uric acid. Stress increases the metabolism and is a common trigger of gout attacks. Avoiding stress is therefore useful in gout.

Deep-breathing exercises are an important prelude to relaxation, excellent for achieving and maintaining overall health, and can be invaluable in reducing the intense pain of a flare-up of gout. Meditation has been shown in research to help normalize blood pressure and boost the immune system, both of which are of great benefit to people with gout.

Deep breathing

In normal breathing, we take oxygen from the atmosphere down into our lungs. The diaphragm contracts, and air is pulled into the chest cavity. When we breathe out, we expel carbon dioxide and other waste gases back into the atmosphere. But when we are stressed or upset, we tend to use the rib muscles to expand the chest. We breathe more quickly, sucking in shallowly. This is good in a crisis as it allows us to obtain the optimum amount of oxygen in the shortest possible time, providing our bodies with the extra power needed to handle the emergency.

Some people do tend to get stuck in chest-breathing mode. Long-term shallow breathing is not only detrimental to our physical and emotional health, it can also lead to hyperventilation, panic attacks, chest pains, dizziness and gastro-intestinal problems.

To test your breathing, ask yourself:

- How fast are you breathing as you are reading this?
- Are you pausing between breaths?
- Are you breathing with your chest or with your diaphragm?

A breathing exercise

The following deep-breathing exercise should, ideally, be performed daily:

1 Make yourself comfortable, either sitting or lying, in a warm room where you know you will be alone for at least half an hour.
2 Close your eyes and try to relax.
3 Gradually slow down your breathing, inhaling and exhaling as evenly as possible.
4 Place one hand on your chest and the other on your abdomen, just below your ribcage.
5 As you inhale, allow your abdomen to swell outwards (your chest should barely move).
6 As you exhale, let your abdomen flatten.

Give yourself a few minutes to get into a smooth, easy rhythm. As worries and distractions arise, don't hang on to them. Wait calmly for them to float out of your mind – then focus once more on your breathing.

When you feel ready to end the exercise, open your eyes. Allow yourself time to become alert before rolling on to one side and getting up. With practice, you will begin breathing with your diaphragm quite naturally – and in times of stress you should be able to correct your breathing without too much effort.

A relaxation exercise

Relaxation is one of the forgotten skills in today's hectic world. We already know that stress – which can give rise to muscle tension, insomnia, hypertension and depression – is one of the greatest enemies of the gout patient. It is advisable, therefore, to learn at least one relaxation technique. The following exercise is perhaps the easiest:

1 Make yourself comfortable in a place where you will not be disturbed – listening to restful music may help you relax.
2 Begin to slow down your breathing, inhaling through your nose to a count of one, two – ensuring that the abdomen pushes outwards, as explained.
3 Exhale to a count of one, two, three, four – or up to five and six.
4 After a couple of minutes, concentrate on each part of the body in turn, starting with your right arm. Consciously relax each set of muscles, allowing the tension to flow right out. Let your arm feel heavier and heavier as every last remnant of tension seeps away. Follow this procedure with the muscles of your left arm, then the muscles of your face, your neck, your stomach, your hips and finally your legs.

Visualization

When you have achieved step four of the relaxation exercise, a technique called visualization can be introduced. As you continue to breathe slowly and evenly, imagine yourself surrounded, perhaps, by lush, peaceful countryside, beside a gently trickling stream – or maybe on a deserted tropical beach, beneath swaying palm fronds, listening to the sounds of the ocean, thousands of miles from your worries and cares. Let the warm sun, the gentle breeze, the peacefulness of it all wash over you.

The tranquillity you feel at this stage can be enhanced by frequently repeating the exercise – once or twice a day is best. With time, you should be able to switch into a calm state of mind whenever you feel stressed.

Meditation

Arguably the oldest natural therapy, meditation is the simplest and most effective form of self-help. Dr Herbert Benson of the Harvard Medical School has been able to show that meditation tends to normalize blood pressure, the pulse rate and the level of stress hormones in the blood. He has also proved that it produces changes in brainwave patterns, which show less excitability, and that it improves the white blood cell (immune) response as well as hormone response. It must therefore be considered an important and easily accessible aid to recovery for people who suffer from gout.

The unusual thing about meditation is that it involves letting go, allowing the mind to roam freely. However, as most of us are used to endeavouring to control our thoughts – in our work, for example – letting go is not as easy as it sounds.

It may help to know that people who regularly meditate say they have more energy, require less sleep, are less anxious and feel far more alive than before they did so. Ideally, the technique should be imparted by a teacher – but as meditation is essentially performed alone, it can be learnt alone with equal success.

Meditation may, to some people, sound a bit offbeat. But isn't it worth a try – especially when you can do it for free? Kick off those shoes and make yourself comfortable, somewhere you can be alone for a while. Now follow these simple instructions:

1 Close your eyes, relax, and practise the deep-breathing exercise as described.
2 Concentrate on your breathing. Try to free your mind of conscious control. Letting it roam unchecked, try to allow the deeper, more serene part of you to take over.
3 If you wish to go further into meditation, concentrate now on mentally repeating a mantra – a certain word or phrase. It should be something positive, such as 'relax', 'I feel calm', 'I am feeling much better' or even 'I am special'.

4 When you are ready to finish, open your eyes and allow yourself time to adjust to the outside world before getting to your feet.

The aim of mentally repeating a mantra is to plant the positive thought into your subconscious mind. It is a form of self-hypnosis, but you alone control the messages placed in your mind.

Mineral tissue salts

Mineral tissue salts therapy is an offshoot of homeopathy and thus completely safe. As with most complementary therapies, this one can be used in conjunction with conventional medication without any side effects. Mineral tissue salts are reputed to be of particular benefit where the body is overly acidic, as is the case for people with gout. They are also useful for treating minor illnesses, from skin conditions to sinus disorders.

The original 12 remedies were isolated by Dr Wilhelm Schuessler in 1880. The natural ingredients are homeopathically prepared to a potency that is reputed to allow the cells to rebalance their salts content, to restore health. The tiny white tablets dissolve in the mouth, leaving a pleasant taste. There are more than 30 different tissue salts in all, but the most useful for gout patients are No. 10 Nat. Phos (sodium phosphate) and, for use during an attack of gout on account of its inflammatory properties, No. 4 Ferr. Phos (iron phosphate). Before you start a course of tissue salts, make sure you read the label instructions.

Mineral tissue salts are available from healthfood shops and chemists.

Reflexology

Reflexology, an ancient oriental therapy, has only recently been adopted in the West. It operates on the proposition that the body is divided into different energy zones, all of which can be exploited in the prevention and treatment of any disorder. Reflexologists have identified ten energy channels, beginning in the toes and extending to the fingers and the top of the head. Each channel relates to a particular bodily zone and to the organs in that zone. For example, the big toe relates to the head – the brain, sinus area, neck, pituitary glands, eyes and ears. By applying pressure to the appropriate terminal in the form of a small, specialized massage, a practitioner can determine which energy pathways are blocked.

Experts in this type of manipulative therapy claim that all the organs of the body are reflected in the feet. They also believe that reflexology aids the removal of waste products and blockages within the energy channels, improving circulation and gland function. Reflexology is certainly relaxing. Indeed, many patients fall asleep during the therapy. Because my own feet are so ticklish, I felt I had cause to worry before my first reflexology session (I could imagine myself involuntarily kicking the therapist). Fortunately, I quickly found that the sensations were pleasurable and I was able to relax – and I must say I was surprised to note how accurate the therapist was in detecting my own indispositions.

Therapists certainly do exert pressure on the tiny crystalline deposits of uric acid that we all have on our feet. However, the idea that the deposits are broken up by reflexology and absorbed into the body's waste disposal system is a matter for debate. The crystals of uric acid present in gout are manifestations of a physical problem experienced by the body rather than within the energy field.

Many therapists prefer to take down a full case history before commencing treatment. Each session will take up to 45 minutes (the preliminary session will take longer), and you will be treated either sitting in a chair or lying down, depending on the therapist and on the patient's condition. There is much ongoing research into the effectiveness of reflexology on arthritic conditions. In fact, it has been known for patients to reduce the intake of cortisone drugs – with their physician's consent, of course – following a course of reflexology treatment.

6

Emotional help

Gout can affect every area of your life. In the early stages of the illness, those with gout are often beset by fears for the future, concerns about the effectiveness of the medications they are prescribed and anxieties about their ability to alter their diet and lifestyle. They are likely even to feel anger over the way gout is viewed by the general public – or even worse, by their families and friends. These factors can be major sources of upset. However, given time, education and self-awareness training, people with gout can gradually come to terms with the condition, finding ways to cope effectively with the stress, the reactions of others and any further outbreaks of pain.

A chronic illness

Even when people with gout are doing all within their power to control the condition – and doing it with success – they will always be predisposed to developing it again. Once gout has reared its ugly head, it sits in the shadows, just waiting to leap out should you put a foot wrong. For this reason, gout is considered a chronic condition, just like all arthritic disease.

It's an unfortunate fact that chronic illness creates a plethora of negative emotions. These emotions are discussed below.

I feel so angry!

When you learn that the searing pain is likely to return, that you must now make permanent and drastic changes to your life, you may feel very angry. After all, your friends are able to continue to enjoy a few beers at the pub, they can eat as much meat as they like, and they haven't been told to lose weight – forgive me if these are not your particular problems, but I'm sure you see what I mean. If it is kidney disease that has brought about your gout, or even medications for another health problem, then that could easily be another cause of anger. After all, you are suffering from one disorder already – it doesn't seem fair that it should have led to another.

It may help to know that anger is a natural response to the diagnosis of chronic disease, and that it is generally followed by acceptance – albeit grudging. I'm afraid the only way to get on top of this illness is to take positive action. It distracts attention from any negative emotions and gives a clear focus.

I feel so afraid!

Of course you feel afraid when you develop an illness for which there is, as yet, no safe and absolute cure. Fears tend to centre around the future, and what will become of you. You may be afraid of repeated attacks; afraid that they will be more painful each time; afraid of the long-term effects of medication; afraid to tell people of the nature of your illness; afraid of being laughed at; afraid of being unable to make the necessary changes to your diet and lifestyle – the list goes on.

There is no doubt that chronic illness exerts a profound effect on the individual. However, most people with gout will say that the fear of the unknown abates with time. They learn that they can still take great pleasure from family life, enjoy social occasions, take up interests and hobbies and be of use to others. Most importantly, people with gout learn that their condition really can be controlled with a little self-determination and the support of their family and friends.

I feel so confused!

After a diagnosis of gout it is common to feel confused. Your doctor may have mentioned medications, but you may be baffled about which you should take, and about their long-term effects. You are likely even to be confused about what steps you need to take to help normalize your hyperuricemia. There is so much to absorb in the early days, especially if you are keen to do what you can to help yourself. You may rest assured, however, that your doctor will know which medications are most suited to your particular needs, and that he or she will be able to guide you through any diet and lifestyle changes you wish to try. It's always helpful to gather together as much information as possible about your condition – from your doctor, pharmacist, bookshop, library and the Internet. It will all help clarify matters. Then take it one step at a time.

I feel so vulnerable!

Vulnerability is a natural human condition. We all need people to love us; we all crave the affirmation of others. To a large extent we are all dependent upon others, measuring their responses in order to reassure ourselves that we are worthwhile human beings, that we are indeed loveable. When an individual has an illness that is perceived as unglamorous and brought about by overindulgence, it can be easy to feel unattractive, unappealing and even greedy. It is even possible to feel no longer loveable.

Feelings of vulnerability will always be present in chronic illness, but to a large extent they can be defeated by looking less to outsiders for affirmation. We all have inner strengths and particular talents, even some of which we may at first be unaware. Yet if we waited for others to point them out we would probably be waiting for ever! Your particular forte may lie in planning and organizing, or problem solving or handling finances – not necessarily out of the family setting. You may be an authority on steam engines, a good listener, a talented artist, an excellent singer, a diligent student, a competent driver – the possibilities are endless. Do not underestimate yourself!

Remember, too, that the people who love you will not stop

doing so because you are living with gout. Love is about who you are – your character and personality, your strengths and weaknesses – your *inner* self.

I feel so guilty!

Feelings of guilt are common in chronic illness. It is natural to want to lay the blame for falling ill at someone's door, and many sufferers imagine they themselves must have done something wrong to deserve such retribution. But blaming either yourself or others is pointless. Life is a lottery. Some people are rich, some poor; some clever, some not so clever; some fall ill, some remain healthy. That's just the way it is.

You may, after learning that improvement lies mainly in your hands, feel guilty about making no real progress. But assuming you have tried to help yourself, there is probably a sound reason for your failure. For example, you may be held back by additional health problems, or you may not have allowed sufficient time for any improvements to show.

I can't accept that I have a chronic disease!

Refusal to accept the needs of the condition is unfortunately very common – but again, it is a very natural response. After a first flare-up and a diagnosis of gout, it can be easy to believe that there will be no recurrence, that it will all go away. I have even come across people who have experienced several attacks and still blithely believe that each is the last. Unfortunately, attacks of gout will always recur if nothing is done to improve the situation. Not only that, the attacks will become increasingly painful and likely to spread to further areas. The knock-on effects of untreated gout attacks can be kidney disease, high blood pressure and heart disease, as already explained.

In my research, it has also become clear that a number of gout sufferers refuse to make the necessary changes to their diet and lifestyle. They have eaten meat and drunk beer all their lives and have no intention of changing now. It's as if they have an impenetrable field around them that will protect them from future health risks. I'm afraid it doesn't quite work that way.

Dealing with other people

The reactions of others can be one of the most difficult aspects of gout. As I noted at the beginning of this book, in the past the condition was ridiculed mercilessly and the general public was left in no doubt that overindulgence was the cause. So how do you cope when the people around you poke fun at you, when they only laugh and tell you you've brought it on yourself? Read on and you will hopefully find some answers.

How can I make people take my condition seriously?

Without doubt, some people are incredibly insensitive. You may feel that you are always on your guard, dreading the remark that will send you into a whirl of anger or the depths of despair. Sadly, developing a condition like gout lays you open to the preconceptions of others. You really should not have to grin and bear the sniggers, the hurtful remarks. Instead, it would be best to try to tell the person, very calmly, that gout is exceedingly painful and no laughing matter.

Standing up for yourself is not easy, but doing so can have a releasing effect – unlike when you fake indifference or clam up and walk away. In such instances, you may end up feeling hurt, offended and very resentful. Your most intense feeling, however, will probably be anger – at the other person and at yourself, for allowing yourself to be hurt.

Dealing with others

It is generally when a person first announces that they have gout that they face the worst of the hurtful remarks. To counter that, it is probably best to arm yourself with as much information on the subject as possible, so you can show them that gout is a serious matter. If the joking continues, it is important for your self-esteem that you tackle those responsible more firmly. For instance, if someone close to you says, 'You must really be living it up – no wonder you've got gout!' you could reply something like, 'Actually, I'm trying very hard to follow the recommended diet – but it isn't easy.' They may reply jokingly that you can't be trying very hard, to which you might reply, 'I'm trying as hard as I can. As a matter of fact I would appreciate some support from you in this – gout isn't an easy condition to conquer.' They will probably really start to listen at this point, which gives you the chance to explain any difficulties you're having.

A condition like gout is much easier to handle when you have the support of your family and friends. However, there may always be some people who fail to see past the old stigma and continue to chuckle at the mention of the word gout. In cases like this, it is best to try to harden your heart to those people. It is their misfortune to possess an inflexible mind – and to have lost your respect.

Self-talk

The way we speak to ourselves has great bearing on our stress levels – and as already stated, stress is a common trigger of attacks of gout. When we analyse our thoughts, we are often surprised at their negativity – but they must be examined before we can begin to change their destructive pattern. When the TV breaks down, for example, your initial thoughts may be, 'It's so unfair! I was really looking forward to watching that film!' 'This is all I need! I can't afford a new set!' 'If the set can be repaired, it will probably cost a small fortune!' 'What am I supposed to do with my time – sit twiddling my thumbs?' Stress-provoking thoughts by any standard!

By being aware that negative thoughts create stress, you

can train yourself into more positive self-talk. Using the same example, you may, instead, think: 'I'll ring around for quotes in the morning – maybe it won't cost much to repair.' 'It was on its last legs anyway – I'll take the opportunity to buy a more up-to-date set.' 'I could buy a new set by paying in instalments.' 'I could buy a reconditioned set if I can't afford a new one.' 'I could borrow one from a friend and not have to worry about repair costs.' 'In the meantime, this is my chance to read that book, to finish my tapestry, to phone Aunt Betty.'

The following examples of stress-relieving self-talk can be applied to many potentially stressful situations:

> 'I'll break this problem into separate sections – they'll be easier to handle.'
> 'I'll take things one step at a time.'
> 'Is this really worth getting upset and angry over?'
> 'I've coped before, so I'll cope again.'
> 'I can always ask for help if I need it.'
> 'It could have been much worse.'
> 'This is hardly a matter of life or death!'
> 'There's nothing I can do about this situation, so I'll have to accept it.'

Lifestyle measures to help prevent gout

Here, in brief, is a reminder of the lifestyle measures necessary for lowering uric acid levels and correcting hyperuricemia:

- Cut down on foods containing purines – meat, poultry and fish (particularly organ meat and shellfish), gravies, asparagus, cauliflower and so on.
- Beware of different eating and drinking patterns, for example on holiday. Before travelling, ask your doctor to prescribe a medication that can be taken at the first sign of gout. In most cases, this will stop the episode in its tracks.
- Try to eat half a dozen cherries every day.
- Take the recommended supplements.

- Maintain a healthy weight – avoid crash dieting.
- Drink plenty of water.
- Cut down on your alcohol consumption.
- Avoid joint injury, if at all possible.
- Avoid stress.

Action for acute attacks

Flare-ups of pain are an ever-present risk in gout. They can be caused by:

- injury to an area affected by gout in the past – a stubbed toe, for example;
- a sharp increase in alcohol consumption;
- surgery;
- illness;
- an infection;
- eating more purine foods than normal;
- not eating enough food (starvation);
- not drinking enough water;
- use of certain prescription drugs.

The following pointers should help you to cope with an attack:

1 Take action as soon as you recognize that an attack is occurring. This may include immediate rest, alternate heat and cold application, painkilling medication – even sending someone out to the shop to buy you some cherries. Remember that you should eat or drink no high-purine foods once an attack is under way. A therapeutic diet – for the duration of the attack – should come largely from cheese, milk, eggs and low-purine vegetables.

2 Be positive! A positive frame of mind can speed recovery. Tell yourself, 'I'll get through this just as I have before.' 'I am more aware of how to help myself this time.' 'I'll make

efforts to distract myself from the pain.' 'I won't let myself get depressed – that will do me more harm than good.'

3 Explore the possible reasons for the increase in pain. Ask yourself, 'Did I eat too much food that contains purines; did I drink too much alcohol?' Maybe in an effort to lose weight you have not been eating enough?

4 Decide how you can reduce the risk of future flare-ups. If you know where you went wrong, take steps to avoid doing so in future.

5 Review the effectiveness of your current flare-up strategy. Are your present medications adequate in a crisis? Is it time to visit your doctor again? Can you do anything further to stay positive? Could you try a new type of complementary therapy?

Useful addresses

Arthritis Care
18 Stephenson Way
London NW1 2HD
Tel.: 020 7380 6500
Helpline: 0808 800 4050
Website: www.arthritiscare.org.uk

There are local and regional offices; a newspaper, *Arthritis News*, is free to members. Free booklets and leaflets may be downloaded from the website.

Arthritis Foundation
PO Box 7669
Atlanta
GA 30357-0669
USA.
Tel.: 1 800 283 7800
Website: www.arthritis.org

Arthritis Research UK (formerly **Arthritis Research Campaign**)
Copeman House
St Mary's Gate
Chesterfield
Derbyshire S41 7TD
Tel.: 01246 558033
Website: www.arthritisresearchuk.org

As well as funding research, this organization produces a range of free information booklets and leaflets.

Al-Anon (England)
61 Great Dover Street
London SE1 4YF
Tel.: 020 7407 0215
Confidential Helpline: 020 7403 0888 (10 a.m. to 10 p.m., 365 days a year)
Website: www.al-anonuk.org.uk

Family groups provide understanding, strength and hope to anyone whose life is, or has been, affected by someone else's drinking. There are other Al-Anon information centres in Ireland and Scotland.

Al-Anon (Northern Ireland)
Al-Anon Information Centre
Peace House
224 Lisburn Road
Belfast BT9 6GE
Tel.: 028 9068 2368 (helpline, 10 a.m. to 1 p.m., Monday to Friday; 6 p.m. to 11 p.m., Monday to Sunday inclusive)

Al-Anon (Republic of Ireland)
Al-Anon Information Centre
Room 5, 5 Capel Street
Dublin 1
Tel.: 01 873 2699 (helpline, 10.30 a.m. to 2.30 p.m., Monday to Friday)

Al-Anon (Scotland)
Al-Anon Information Centre
Mansfield Park Building, Unit 6
22 Mansfield Street
Partick
Glasgow G11 5QP
Tel.: 0141 339 8884 (helpline, 10 a.m. to 10 p.m., 365 days a year)

Association of Reflexologists
5 Fore Street
Taunton
Somerset TA1 1HX
Tel.: 01823 351010
Website: www.aor.org.uk

British Acupuncture Council
63 Jeddo Road
London W12 9HQ
Tel.: 020 8735 0400 (9.30 a.m. to 5.30 p.m., Monday to Friday)
Website: www.acupuncture.org.uk

British Homeopathic Association
Hahnemann House
29 Park Street West
Luton LU1 3BE
Tel.: 01582 408675
Website: www.britishhomeopathic.org

Cherry Active Ltd
99 Manor Lane
Sunbury
Middlesex TW16 6JE
Tel.: 01932 706881
Website: www.cherryactive.co.uk

A commercial organization providing cherry-juice products and advice on the benefits of cherries in the treatment of gout and arthritis.

Magnets for All
The Old Laundry
Dauntsey Park
Dauntsey
Chippenham
Wilts SN15 4HT
Tel.: 01249 721482
Website: www.magnetsforall.com

Distributors of Bioflow personal magnetic-therapy items.

NHS Direct
Tel.: 0845 46 47
Website: www.nhsdirect.nhs.uk

The Nutri Centre
Unit 3, Kendal Court
Kendal Avenue
London W3 0RU
Tel.: 0845 602 6744 (mail order and general enquiries); if calling from outside the UK, 00 44 845 602 6744. Mail order opening hours: 9 a.m. to 6 p.m., Monday to Friday; 10 a.m. to 4 p.m., Saturday.
Website: www.nutricentre.com

Provides details of nutritional products and complementary medicines which may be bought through their online store. The site also provides details of shops in the UK that stock their products.

Synergy
44 Caskie Drive
Blantyre G72 9XG
Tel.: 01698 827335
Website: www.synergy-health.co.uk

You can email Synergy from the website to obtain information about the Hay food combining system.

UK Gout Society
PO Box 527
London WC1V 7YP
Website: www.ukgoutsociety.org

Vanderbell Health
Vanderbell Publishing Ltd
59 Capital Business Centre
22 Carlton Road
Croydon CR2 0BS
24-hour order line: 020 8916 2111
Website: www.health4youonline.com

Vanderbell Health supplies petrochemical-free MSM.

Weight Watchers (UK) Ltd
Millennium House
Ludlow Road
Maidenhead
Berkshire SL6 2SL
Website: www.weightwatchers.co.uk

For details of Weight Watchers meetings in the UK, write to the address
above or refer to the website.

References

1   P. Thiehle and H.E. Schroder, 'Epidemiology and pathogenesis of disorders of purine metabolism', *Ter Arkh*, 1997, 59 (4), pp. 14–18.
2   H.R. Schumacher Jr, J.A. Boice, D.I. Daikj et al., 'Randomized double-blind trial of etoricoxib and indometacin in the treatment of acute gouty arthritis', *BMJ* 2, 2002, 324, pp. 1488–92.
3   'Cherry diet control for gout and arthritis', *Texas Reports on Biology and Medicine* V8, Fall 1950.
4   *The McDougall Program: Twelve days to dynamic health*, NAL Books, 1990, p. 312.
5   Wayne State University College of Medicine – reported in *Better Nutrition*, March 1990, 52 (3), p. 9.
6   Cass et al. *Geriatrics*, 1954, 9, p. 375.
7   X. Liu, L. Sun, J. Xiao, S. Yin, C. Liu, Q. Li, H. Li and B. Jin, 'Effect of acupuncture and point-injection treatment on immunologic function in rheumatoid arthritis', General Hospital of PLA, Beijing, *Journal of Traditional Chinese Medicine*, September 1993, 13 (3), pp. 174–8.
8   I.N. Ruchkin and A.P. Burdeinyl, 'Auriculo-electropuncture in rheumatoid arthritis (a double-blind study)', *Ter Arkh*, 1987, 59 (12), pp. 26–30.
9   B.B. Domangue, C.G. Margolis, D. Lieberman and H. Kaji, 'Biochemical correlates of hypnoanalgesia in arthritic pain patients', *Journal of Clinical Psychiatry*, June 1985, 46 (6), pp. 235–8.

Further reading

Penny Doyle and Audrey Deane, *The Top 100 Omega-3 Recipes: Reduce your risk of heart disease, keep your brain active and agile*, Duncan Baird Publishers, 2009.

Bryan Emmerson, *Getting Rid of Gout*, Oxford University Press, 2003.

Rodney Grahame et al., *Gout – The 'At Your Fingertips Guide'*, Class Publishing, 2003.

Louise Hagler, *Tofu Cookery: 25th anniversary edition*, Book Publishing Company, 2008.

Leslie and Susannah Kenton, *The Raw Energy Bible*, Vermilion, 2001.

Victor Konshin, *Beating Gout: A sufferer's guide to living pain free*, Ayerware Publishing, 2009.

Ronald Melzack and Patrick D. Wall, *The Challenge of Pain* (Penguin Science), Penguin, 2008.

Andrew Weil, *Eating Well for Optimum Health: The essential guide to food, diet and nutrition*, Sphere, 2008.

Index

CPSIA information can be obtained at www.ICGtesting.com
Printed in the USA
LVOW100957030613

336655LV00015B/292/P

9 781847 091482